1000

ISQs for the

MRCPsych

S Rajarathinam, MBBS, DPM, MD
Assistant Professor and Consultant Psychiatrist
Stanley Medical College Hospital.
Chennai, India.

S Rajagopal, MBBS, DPM (Ireland), MRCPsych
Consultant Psychiatrist
South London & Maudsley NHS Trust
St Thomas' Hospital
London

Lena Kathiravan Palaniyappan
        BA (Psych), MBBS, PGDPsyCouns
Senior House Officer (FLOAT)
Maudsley Hospital
South London and Maudsley NHS Trust
Denmark Hill
London

Paras Medical Publisher
Solutions for Health Care Professionals

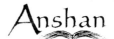

To
Our parents, Theo, Vasanth and Archana

1000 ISQs for the MRCPsych

First published in the UK by

ANSHAN LTD
In 2006

6 Newlands Road, Tunbridge Wells,
Kent. TN4 9AT. UK
Tel/Fax: +44 (0) 1892 557767
e-mail: info@anshan.co.uk
Web Site: www.anshan.co.uk

Published in arrangement with
Paras Medical Publisher, 5-1-475 First Floor
Putlibwoli, Hyderabad - 500 095, India.
E-mail: parasmedpub@hotmail.com

© S Rajarathinam, Lena Kathiravan P, S Rajagopal

ISBN 10: 1 904 79887 X
ISBN 13: 978 1 904798 87 3

Note: As new information becomes available, changes become necessary. The editors/authors/contributors and the publishers have, as far as it is possible, taken care to ensure that the information given in this book is accurate and up-to-date. In view of the possibility of human error or advances in medical science neither the editor nor the publisher nor any other party who has been involved in the preparation or publication of this work warrants that the information contained herein is in every respect accurate or complete. Readers are encouraged to consult standard references.

British Library Cataloguing in Publication Data
A catalogue record for this book is available from the British Library

Preface

We cannot help but think the famous words of Samuel Butler when we start preparing for the MRCPsych ISQs –

"Life is a process of drawing sufficient conclusions from insufficient premises"!

Of course we fully well agree that for many of our breed, MRCPsych is no smaller than life. **"To talk of diseases is a sort of Arabian Nights entertainment"**, says Sir William Osler. But we are sure that he did not talk through the ISQ language anyway. So how should we go about tackling this? Let us take the bull by its horns!

We believe that more than the immense load of facts that is demanded for successful victory over ISQs, noting the subtle and tactful ways of stating the question will help in sweeping a decent score. This needs a lot of practice. Needless to say, you need a treasury of finely crafted and carefully carved ISQs to keep the momentum going. That is exactly what you have here!! Please provide us with your valuable suggestions and criticism. We really need them. Also don't forget to convey the message of your success.

Wishing you all the best,

Rajarathinam S
S Rajagopal
Lena Kathiravan Palaniyappan

Acknowledgements

But for our patients this book would not be here—We pray for you. But for our parents we would not be here—We love you.

We thank our teachers and mentors who inspired us into this eternal field of Psychiatry. We stand grateful to one great institution which links us—Stanley Medical College and Hospital, Chennai.

Our special thanks to Mr Divyesh Kothari, who offered his full fledged support and immediate acceptance to publish this book.

Contents

Basic Neurosciences

Questions

1. All or none law does not hold good for axoaxonal synapses.

2. Conjoint synapses are multineuronal units.

3. Long term potentiation (LTP) is the strengthening of synapses by repeated coordinated neuronal activity.

4. Cholinergic neurotransmission occurs through tyrosine kinase intermediation.

5. Adenosine is a neurotransmitter.

6. Excitotoxicity kills the presynaptic neuron before the postsynaptic neuronal death.

7. All excitatory amino acid neurotransmitters are monocarboxylic amino acids.

8. Nicotine reduces glutamate release.

Answers

....

1.   True

2.   False: They are combined electrochemical synapses.

3.   True: LTP is the cellular correlate of long term memory.

4.   False: Cholinergic Muscarinic–G protein coupled; Nicotinic–
     Ligand gated ion channels.

5.   True: Adenosine is a minor neurotransmitter. P_1 receptors
     are the adenosine receptors, blocked by xanthine, with two
     subgroups A_1 and A_2. Adenosine is released during seizure
     activity and it inhibits all neurotransmitters nonselectively.

6.   False: Excitotoxicity, mediated by NMDA-glutamate, Ca^{2+} and
     NO, has a self-sparing effect.

7.   False: Monocorboxylic acids are inhibitory and dicarboxylic
     acids are excitatory.

8.   False: Nicotine increases glutamate release–can be utilized
     to treat some side effects of haloperidol.

Questions

9. NMDA receptor needs three neurotransmitter molecules to get activated.

10. Remacemide is a NMDA inhibitor.

11. Glycine is always inhibitory.

12. Activation of D_2 receptors inhibits caudate function.

13. Peptide neurotransmitters have only 100 to 200 amino acids.

14. Somatostatin levels are increased in both Huntington's and Alzheimer's disease.

15. The sole source of human melatonin is pineal-hypothalamus system.

Answers

....

9.   True: Two glutamates – one glycine molecules

10.   True

11.   False: Non strychnine sensitive receptors are excitatory.

12.   True

13.   False: Only 2-40 AA are present.

14.   False: Increased in Huntington's; reduced in Alzheimer's.

15.   False: Retinal photoreceptors produce melatonin locally.

16. The duration of human circadian cycle is the same as normal day-night cycle.

17. Variations noted in 5-HT reuptake channel structure can explain trait anxiety.

18. GABA plays a vital role in homunculus formation.

19. Acetylcholine is the chief neurotransmitter identified in alcohol withdrawal delirium.

20. Senile plaques of amyloid are noted in lead encephalopathy.

21. Loss of 50 mL of brain volume leads to moderate–severe dementia.

22. Acute intermittent porphyria is due to ALA[1] synthetase deficiency.

23. Hypofrontality is characteristic of schizophrenia.

1 ALA – Amino Levulanic Acid

Answers

16. False: The circadian cycle is 24.5 hours in duration on average

17. True

18. False: Serotonin is more important. Defective homunculus formation is seen in Williams's syndrome.

19. False: Though acetylcholine is the defective transmitter in most cases of delirium, increased norepinephrine in locus ceruleus is suspected to cause delirium tremens.

20. True: It is seen in CJD, Down's and normal aging, apart from Alzheimer's.

21. False: 50 mL loss leads to mild cognitive impairment. 100 ml loss leads to dementia.

22. False: It is due to hydroxy methyl bilane synthase deficiency.

23. False: It is not universal in Schizophrenia itself. Further it is seen in major depression also.

24. Auditory hallucination can be explained by genetically determined reduced response to noise in some.

25. Gamma hydroxyl butyrate (liquid ecstasy) acts via opioid system.

26. Monosodium glutamate is panicogenic.

27. Endocrine dysfunction in the form of increased cortisol levels is seen in Chronic Fatigue Syndrome.

28. Genomic imprinting disorders decrease with assisted reproductive techniques.

29. Growth promoting genes are usually paternally imprinted.

30. Fragile X syndrome occurs only in males.

31. DNPH[2] test is used in detecting PKU.

2 DNPH – Di Nitro Phenyl Hydrazine

Answers

24. False: It should be excessive response to noise.

25. True It can cause pseudo Wernicke-Korsakoff syndrome.

26. True. Its presence in Chinese foods causes Chinese restaurant syndrome.

27. False: Hypocortisolemia is noted

28. False: Assisted reproduction increases incidence of genomic imprinting

29. True

30. False: Xq27.3 CGG repeat occurs in both sexes

31. False: It is employed in maple syrup urine disease.

Questions

32. Right left differentiation in a visual stimulus is perceived by right parietal (non dominant) lobe.

33. Place code or navigation map is formed in hippocampus.

34. Right frontal seizure activity produces gelastic seizures.

35. *Aplysia california* is a snail model of anxiety.

36. Neurochemical panicogens act on nucleus paragigantocellularis and baroreceptors.

37. Among phobias, blood-injection-injury type is the least heritable.

38. In short sleepers NREM sleep is markedly reduced

39. Transition to REM sleep occurs from stage 4 normally.

Answers

....

32. True: Contour perception occurs in right lobe. Left perceives complex inner details.

33. True

34. False: Left frontal seizures produces spells of laughter, gelastic seizures

35. True

36. True

37. False: Unlike other phobias it is strongly heritable, associated with bradycardia and hypotension.

38. False: NREM period is normal while REM is shortened.

39. False: Stage 1-2-3-4-3-2-REM-2-3-4-3-2-REM...is the normal cycling process, each cycle from stage 1 to post REM stage2 lasting 90 minutes.

40. Hypocretin is identified as the neurochemical involved in narcolepsy.

41. Somniloquy occurs in stage 4 sleep.

42. High sociability and MAO levels are negatively correlated.

43. EEG abnormalities consistent with minimal brain damage are common in antisocial personality disorder.

44. Abnormal DST is demonstrated in schizoid personality disorder.

45. Confabulation in amnesic disorders is a sign of parietal damage.

46. Procedural memory is intact in transient global amnesia.

Answers

40. True: It is also called Orexin

41. True. It can occur at any stage

42. True

43. True

44. False: It is seen in borderline personalities.

45. False: Frontal involvement is suspected.

46. True: These patients can drive without knowing where they are heading.

47. Interictal psychosis is more common in left handed females especially around puberty.

48. MAO is a mitochondrial enzyme.

49. Pyridostigmine produces growth hormone surge in OCD patients.

50. Retina and olfactory bulb have long acting dopamine tracts.

51. Liddle's disorganization syndrome is due to bilateral parietal and anterior cingulate pathology.

52. Novelty seeking is mapped on to chromosome 17

53. Polymicrogyria and hypoplastic vermis are noted in ADHD

54. Zinc deficiency can cause a craving for ice.

55. Locus ceruleus is called the behavioural pacemaker.

Answers

47. True

48. True

49. True

50. False: They have ultra short acting dopamine tracts.

51. True: Reality distortion is due to left medial temporal pathology. Frontal involvement causes psychomotor poverty.

52. False: It is related to chromosome 11, while neuroticism is linked to 17.

53. False: They are seen in autism.

54. True: This variant of pica is similar to dirt craving in iron deficiency.

55. False: Raphe nucleus enjoys this privilege.

56. Exaggerated response to tropicamide in pupillary dilatation is noted in Alzheimer's disease.

57. Kindling is a behavioural technique of inducing pseudoseizures.

58. Chromosome X is implicated in catatonic schizophrenia.

59. Theta waves show circadian and menstrual variation.

60. Delta waves can be induced by hyperventilation.

61. P ^{300} is altered in Alzheimer's dementia.

62. Epinephrine is a precursor of norepinephrine.

63. Blood cells show benzodiazepine receptors

64. Compton effect is change in SPECT resolution due to deviation of emitted photons.

Answers

56. True

57. False: Repeated subthreshold stimulation leading to action potential generation, operating in mood disorders possibly, is kindling.

58. False: In bipolar type I.

59. False: α shows such difference.

60. True

61. True: P^{300} is an event related potential, maximum over parietal lobe. It shows reduced amplitude in autism, schizophrenia, Down's and Alzheimer's. In developmental dysphasia the amplitude is increased.

62. False: Norepinephrine when acted upon by PNMT (phenyl ethanolamine N methyl transferase) produces epinephrine.

63. True: They are called acceptors. WBCs, mast cells and platelets have them.

64. True

65. Anatomical resolution is better for PET than SPECT.

66. GABA is implicated in harm avoidance behaviour

67. VTA is a part of limbic system.

68. Raphe nucleus promotes arousal by being a part of ARAS.

69. Episodic memory is a function of limbic system.

70. Lipid substances cannot be neurotransmitters.

71. In a receptor the selective binding site is often the extracellular portion.

72. Leucine zipper is a late gene transcription factor.

73. An antagonist cannot block the actions of an inverse agonist.

74. Excitotoxicity causes panic disorder.

Answers

....

65. True: It is measured by FWHM–Full width at half maximum.

66. True: Dopamine–Novelty seeking; Glutamate–persistence; Noradrenaline and serotonin–reward dependence.

67. False: Periaqueductal gray is the only midbrain limbic structure.

68. False: Locus ceruleus, VTA, cholinergic area 5 and 6 constitute ARAS. Raphe nucleus is a part of proposed ARIS.

69. True

70. False: Anandamide is a lipid neurotransmitter.

71. False: In contrary to popular belief, it is the transmembrane portion.

72. True: It is made of two early gene activation products Fos and Jun.

73. False

74. False: Overexcitation due to too much glutamate mediated Ca^{2+} is demonstrated–but not frank excitotoxic neuronal loss.

75. Locus ceruleus decides whether external or internal focusing of attention is needed at a given time.

76. β_1 receptor regulates mood in noradrenergic projections.

77. Tryptophan is transported into neurons by serotonin reuptake pump.

78. α_2 presynaptic receptors control serotonin release.

79. Non synaptic neurotransmission is seen in substance P pathways.

80. Stimulating α_1 adrenoreceptor may increase serotonin transmission.

81. Tryptophan is the most abundant of free aminoacids in the CNS.

82. Benzodiazepine receptors are abundant in extra CNS sites.

Answers

....

75. True: This later helps in memory formation and learning.

76. True

77. False: Inspite of being the precursor it has its own transport pump.

78. True: α_2 heteroreceptor inhibits both NEN and 5HT release. Apart from this $5HT_{1D}$ and $_{1A}$ are also autoreceptors for serotonin.

79. True: Substance P and its receptor NK_1 are distributed differently, suggesting nonsynaptic volume neurotransmission for substance P.

80. True: α_1 heteroreceptor on 5HT neurons can accelerate 5HT release.

81. False: Glutamate is the mentioned AA.

82. True: Kidney shows w_3 receptor subtype.

83. α$_2$ regulates cognition and attention in noradrenergic projections.

84. Substance P acts on all neurokinin receptors.

85. Stimulating postsynaptic 5HT$_{1A}$ and 5HT$_{2A}$ has opposing effects on mood.

86. In panic disorder.abnormal hemispheric asymmetry is noted in parahippocampal area.

87. 5HT$_{2A}$ stimulation inhibits orgasm.

88. Alprostadil produces arousal even if libido is absent.

89. Galanin is both a hormone and a neurotransmitter.

90. Leptin belongs to IL-6 cytokine family.

91. In anorexia nervosa, leptin levels are low.

Answers

....

83. True

84. False: It acts on NK type I only. Neurokinin A and B act on NK-2 and NK-3.

85. True: $5HT_{1A}$ stimulation elevates mood.

86. True

87. True

88. True: This is not the case with Sildenafil.

89. True: It controls feeding behaviours along with leptin and NP-Y.

90. True

91. True: In obesity leptin levels are high suggesting leptin resistance.

92. CB_1 receptors for endocannabinoids are distributed in the immune cells.

93. CART peptides constitute a neurotransmitter system in drug abuse.

94. M_3 cholinergic receptors are likely candidates in memory functions.

95. Cholinergic agents acting via M1 receptors can modify amyloid processing.

96. Pure D_3 blockade can reduce psychomotor behaviour.

97. Sensory gating deficits in schizophrenia families correlate with α_7 cholinergic receptor defect.

98. CCK-B is the predominant CNS receptor for cholecystokinin.

Answers

....

92. False: CB$_2$ receptors are abundant in immune system.

93. True: CART stands for cocaine and amphetamine related transcript peptides. They have a role in drug abuse and stress induced eating behaviour.

94. False: M$_1$ receptors are the most likely candidates.

95. True: This is a therapeutic advantage in Alzheimer's.

96. False: They increase psychomotor behaviour.

97. True:

98. True: CCK-A is mostly peripheral.

99. In ADHD hyperactivity is mediated via nigrostriatal pathway.

100. Neurotensin is colocalized with dopamine in nigrostriatum.

101. Entorhinal cortex is a transitional cortex.

102. Hippocampal neuronal density is reduced in autism.

103. Locus ceruleus plays a major role in phobic avoidance.

104. Anterior attention system comprises of basal ganglia and DLPFC[3]

105. Anterior cingulate cortex organizes response to pain.

106. Cingulate seizures produce involuntary vocalizations.

3 DLPFC – Dorso Lateral Pre Frontal Cortex

Answers

....

99. True

100. False: This colocalization is selective for mesolimbic pathway only.

101. True: It is 6 layered, still retaining some paleo-cortical organizations.

102. False: It is increased inspite of reduced neuronal size.

103. False: It is important in anticipatory anxiety. Prefrontal cortex mediates avoidance.

104. True

105. True: So cingulotomy is tried as a last resort in chronic pain.

106. True

107. Stutterers show decreased blood flow in left paragenu area.

108. Petalia refers to the asymmetry in size of frontal lobes.

109. Anterior callosal damage is implicated in alien hand sign.

110. Females have larger anterior commissure.

111. Left temporal lobe holds memory of geometric shapes.

112. Frequently crying infants show right frontal activation.

113. Pedunculopontine nucleus regulates pill rolling tremor of Parkinson's disease.

114. Gliosis and cell loss in pallidum correlates with catatonia in schizophrenia.

Answers

....

107. True

108. True: Right lobe is larger usually.

109. True

110. True: That may explain the higher average social intelligence in females.

111. False: Right lobe is responsible for this.

112. True

113. True

114. True

115. In cross fostering design adoptive parent is affected by the disorder.

116. K complex is evoked by internal stimuli only.

117. Microsleep denotes paucity of synaptic transmission.

118. Infants have sleep onset REM period.

119. Stage 2 occupies most of the total sleep time.

120. During sleep mentation all senses are involved in approximate waking state proportions.

121. Septum pellucidum perforations are seen in punch drunk syndrome.

122. Brain ethanol is readily visible using H^1 magnetic resonance spectroscopy.

123. Long term synaptic depression is a cellular correlation of learning.

Answers

....

115. True

116. False: Even external auditory stimuli can evoke K complexes.

117. False: It is a sleep episode less than 30 seconds, occurring in excessive sleepiness.

118. True

119. True: 45–55%

120. True

121. True

122. True

123. True: Like LTP it is also NMDA mediated.

124. Galanin increases carbohydrate preference.

125. Insulin level in CSF is lowered in Alzheimer's.

126. Melatonin intake improves quality and duration of sleep.

127. Paratharmone is a potent analgesic.

128. Olfactory and GnRH neurons migrate along the same pathway during development.

129. Neuropathological insult in Schizophrenia occurs soon after third trimester.

130. Tuberomamillary hypothalamic nucleus contains cell bodies of histaminergic neurons.

131. GABA is present in ß islet cells of pancreas.

132. Taurine levels reach a peak immediately after synaptogenesis.

Answers

....

124. False: It increases fat preference.

125. True

126. True

127. False: It is a hyperalgesic agent.

128. True: So anosmia and hypogonadism occur together in Kallman's syndrome.

129. False: Schizophrenia is one neurodegenerative disease without Gliosis. So any injury should be occurring before third trimester, when glial cells are still non responsive.

130. True

131. True

132. False: Taurine level is high in immature brain. It falls after synaptogenesis. It lacks several properties of a putative neurotransmitter.

133. Alcohol is a negative modulator of glycine neuro transmission.

134. Poly $_A$ tail of RNA carries important genetic information.

135. An abnormality in cortical layer proportion is a feature of William's syndrome.

136. Metabolism in occipital region is spared in Alzheimer's dementia.

137. N acetyl aspartate is restricted to viable neurons.

138. PLIDD[4] are seen in CJD.

139. Triphasic waves are the hallmark of delirium.

140. D_4 are the only subtype of dopamine receptors present in brain stem.

4 PLIDD – Periodic Long Interval Diffuse Discharges

Answers

133. False: It is a positive modulator.

134. False: It serves to simply stabilize the RNA within the cell.

135. True

136. True: But neuritic plaques are frequently demonstrated here.

137. True: It is employed in MRS.

138. False: PSIDD are seen in CJD (short – 0.5 to 1s). PLIDD are seen in SSPE.

139. False: They are mostly seen in delirium due to a metabolic cause.

140. True

141. Posterior parietal seizures produce body image distortions.

142. Insula has a cardiac control center.

143. Primary visual cortex perceives images in linear context.

144. Sleep spindles are subcortical activities.

145. Parietal seizures produce task performance inconsistencies.

146. Tactile imageries are the most common perceptual disturbances in phobia.

147. Balint's syndrome occurs in one sided vascular lesions usually.

Answers

....

141. False: It increases this ratio for sensory signals.

142. True: Phantom limb phenomenon is also noted.

143. True: It has a role on panic related palpitations etc.

144. True

145. True

146. True: This mimics hysteria!!

147. True

148. Movement agnosia is c... to frontal lesions.

149. Movement agnosia is due to frontal lesions.

150. The hippocampus is supplied by the posterior cerebral artery.

Answers

150. True

Psychology

1. Assimilation is taking in of new experiences to existing knowledge system.

2. Curiosity is an important component of secondary circular reactions.

3. Imitation is the first step towards symbolic thought.

4. According to Bowlby, clear-cut attachment occurs in 6 – 24 months.

5. Stranger anxiety develops soon after separation anxiety.

6. Anaclitic depression occurs with attachment failure.

7. Adventitious reinforcement is the accidental pairing of response and reinforcer.

8. Premack's principle is the same as 'grandma's rule'.

Answers

....

1. True: This is a Piagetian concept.

2. False: Cognition is important component in secondary, pleasure in primary and curiosity in tertiary circular reactions.

3. False: Deferred imitation is generally thought of as first step towards symbolic thought.

4. True: From then the baby cries on separation.

5. False: Stranger anxiety develops at 8 months and separation anxiety around 1 year of age.

6. False: According to Rene Spitz it occurs after separation from an established attachment.

7. True: It is said to operate in some phobias.

8. True: "If you eat spinach, you will get a toffee"

9. Festinger proposed cognitive resonance as the disharmony among knowledge, belief and behaviour.

10. Releasers are specific environmental stimuli triggering specific responses.

11. Sensory deprivation reduces suggestibility.

12. Engrossment is a father's initial attachment to the child.

13. Tower of London test measures Basal Ganglia function.

14. Subjective units of distress (SUDS) measures worthlessness.

15. WAIS has more verbal than performance subtests.

16. Time pressure is not applied in Sentence Completion test.

Answers

....

9.   False: It is cognitive dissonance

10.   True: Tinbergen called these 'innate releasing mechanisms'.

11.   False: It increases suggestibility.

12.   True

13.   True

14.   False: It is a unit for phobic items in hierarchy.

15.   True: 6 verbal; 5 performance

16.   False: Time pressure is applied in SCT.

17. Hartmann proposed autonomous ego functions.

18. Fictional finalism is characterized by imaginary motivating ideas with no counterparts in reality.

19. Ocnophilia can follow the perception of 'basic fault'.

20. Holocoenosis is the response in one part of the body to an event in another part.

21. Epinosic gain is the sympathy of caregivers.

22. Ambiguous stimuli promote cognitive organization.

23. Ambiguity in projective tests bypasses conscious awareness and defenses.

24. In structured interview ordering but not the exact wording may be changed.

Answers

17. True

18. True: This is Adler's concept.

19. True: Michael Balint's 'basic fault' is the feeling of something missing in life. It later leads to deep relations (ocnophilia) or aloofness (philobatism).

20. True: Goldstein proposed this.

21. True: Paranosic gain is the direct gain from the illness.

22. False: They produce cognitive disorganization leading to dependence on internal resources to confront them successfully.

23. True: Thus they bring out latent psychopathology.

24. False: Both should be preserved.

25. Binary management means staff and inmates of a mental hospital live in different circumstances.

26. Classical conditioning cannot occur in decorticate specimens.

27. Intermittent reinforcement provides no resistance to extinction.

28. In precontemplation there is a strong intention to change.

29. Imagined flooding can worsen depression.

30. Autonomic arousal to stress is lower in the aged.

31. Narcissism is necessary for deep object relations.

32. Cloninger was a proponent of biosocial model of personality.

Answers

....

25. True: This is one feature of Goffman's "total institutions".

26. False: Even flatworms and decorticate animals demonstrate classical conditioning; the association need not be understood for the reflex response to occur.

27. False: It provides more resistance than the continuous reinforcement.

28. False: There is no intention to change. Precontemplation is the first stage in behavioural change according to MET (Motivational enhancement therapy)

29. True: This CBT technique requires cautious usage.

30. True

31. True

32. True

33. Heredity can explain 60% of individual personality differences.

34. Looping is the collapse of patient's defenses on himself.

35. Openness to experience has the highest hereditary input in the five factor model.

36. Sensation seeking correlates with high platelet MAO activity.

37. Jung introduced active imagination.

38. Wilhelm Reich developed character analysis.

39. Klein claimed a later development of Oedipal complex than what Freud proposed.

Answers

33. False: Studies suggest 40% contribution by heredity. [Loehlin JC (1992) Genes and environment in personality development. Sage, Newbury Park, LA]

34. True: It was coined by Goffman. It happens when his own evidences are used against him in an institutional setup.

35. True: Conscientiousness is the least heredity influenced trait.

36. False: Sensation seeking and impulsivity correlate with low MAO activity.

37. True: It involves encouraging fantasies.

38. True

39. False: She assumed it to develop earlier.

40. Illness behaviour is an innate property of humans.

41. Jung viewed dreams to be compensatory for one sided conscious attitude.

42. Male intelligence is more widely distributed around the mean than the female intelligence.

43. In Likert scale different response patterns can end up with the same score.

44. Simple observation may facilitate the occurrence of certain responses.

45. Attachment begins with representation of mother's face in central retinal field.

46. Fear of heights start at 3 years of age.

Answers

....

40. False: It is usually a learned behaviour.

41. True: This is in sharp contrast to Freudian views.

42. True: So mental retardation may be more common in males.

43. True: This happens with Thurstone scale too.

44. True: This is called the audience effect.

45. False: It starts immediately after birth.

46. False: It begins as early as 6 months.

47. In Klein's schema, infant has an instinctual knowledge of human body.

48. At 6 years of age child fears death more than parental separation.

49. Rebellion is most likely in the late teens.

50. Imprinting applies to all animals except humans.

51. Benton visual retention test provides an impairment index.

52. Following first heart attack survival is better for type A than type B personalities.

53. Annihilation anxiety leads to splitting.

54. Losing job is the most stressful event in Holmes & Rahe scale.

Answers

47. True: So the infant believes that his mother's breast is unavailable when weaning occurs because of father's penis in her vagina.

48. False: Irreversibility of death is understood only after age 8 or 9.

49. False: It is more in early teens.

50. False: Imprinting is clearly demonstrated in some but not all animals, especially primates.

51. False: Halsted Reitan battery yields this score.

52. True: They have a lower chance of a second attack.

53. True: This is a Kleinian concept.

54. False: The death of spouse is the most traumatic event.

55. IQ of older people is less than younger population.

56. Rorschach cannot be used quantitatively.

57. Isolation of affect is the defense behind *la belle indifference.*

58. State dependent learning is absent in humans.

59. Stimulus preparedness acts in almost all phobias.

60. Cognitive Analytical Theory (CAT) was proposed by Aaron Beck.

61. Mirroring is the unconscious imitation of sibling's behaviour.

62. The commonest method attempted to reduce cognitive dissonance is attitudinal change.

Answers

....

55. True: May be due to disparity in educational standards.

56. False: Using Exner scoring method, reliable numerical values can be assigned.

57. True

58. False: It requires very high dose to produce a 'state', but it is seen in humans e.g. amphetamine intoxication.

59. False: According to Seligman, it operates only in selected stimuli that threatened primitive man.

60. False: Anthony Ryle proposed it.

61. False: According to Kohut, this is a safe and positive reflection of the infant's own behaviour and feelings leading to introjection and positive self esteem.

62. False: Behavioural change is more common.

Questions

63. Reduction in conformity pressure needs support from a major faction of the group.

64. Leniency error is the tendency to choose "cannot say" more often than predicted.

65. A sign stimulus elicits a modal action pattern.

66. Imprinting cannot occur outside the critical period.

67. Bronfenbenner proposed ecological systems theory.

68. A not B error is seen in stage 4 of object permanence.

69. Babbling drift hypothesis argues that babbling foreruns language development.

70. Babbling differs in quality among various linguistic groups.

Answers

63.   False: Just one other's dissent is often sufficient to rebel.

64.   False: It is a tendency to select extremes.

65.   True: These are ethological terms. Innate releasing mechanisms (sign stimuli) elicit a chain of responses.

66.   False: It can occur but with great difficulty. So we use 'sensitive period' now.

67.   True: It represents interrelationships of the individual with layers of environmental context.

68.   True: This A not B error is infant's tendency to look for hidden objects in the place last found rather than the place last hidden.

69.   True

70.   False

71. Means and end must be understood to produce intentional behaviour.

72. Babies look at different things for different periods of time.

73. Touch sensitivity develops only after birth.

74. The culture is the nearest microsystem in ecological systems theory.

75. Place learning is learning the specific environmental locations at which reinforcement occurred.

76. Organization is a mnemonic strategy.

77. Piaget employed overt motor behaviours to assess cognitive development.

Answers

....

71. True: This happens between 8–12 months.

72. True: This important observation by Fantz made exploring infant's visual behaviour simpler.

73. False: As early as 2nd month of conception, response to stroking is noted.

74. False: It forms the outermost macrosystem.

75. True

76. True: Rehearsal and elaboration are other strategies.

77. True: This might have caused certain underestimations.

78. Metamemory is the knowledge about memory.

79. Constructive memory operates in building up process only.

80. Robbie Case is a neopiagetian.

81. Operating space refers to the resources necessary to carry out cognitive operations.

82. Automatization helps solving the problem in the practiced but not advanced forms.

83. Transitivity is a formal operational achievement.

84. Abstract thinking is a primary mental ability.

85. Spacing of children affects the intellectual level in a family.

Answers

....

78. True

79. False: It can distort facts too.

80. True: He is an information processing theorist.

81. True

82. False

83. False: This ability to combine relations logically appears in concrete operational development.

84. False: Atleast according to Thurstone.

85. True: This is according to Zajonc's confluence model.

86. More words are spoken than understood at 18 months of age.

87. Overextension is using the same name for various things.

88. Punishment is the most consistent method of obtaining behaviour change.

89. Centration is focusing on what is perceptually ambiguous.

90. Naming explosion occurs at 3 years of age.

91. Babbling is absent in deafness.

92. In first order analysis, few independent personality-defining factors are identified.

93. In repression the reality has never been consciously appreciated.

Answers

86. False: 50 spoken vs. 100 understood on average.

87. True

88. False

89. False: It is focusing on the obvious–characteristic of preoperational child.

90. False: 18 months.

91. False

92. False: This is second order analysis.

93. False: This is denial.

94. Whistling in the dark is denial of fear.

95. Success of training is more dependent on method employed than the child's developmental level.

96. Overregularization is a semantic error.

97. Sex cleavage is the earliest embryological structure in sex differentiation.

98. Adult responses for the same stimulus differ with the assumed sex of the baby.

99. Good co-operation among the children is needed for successful parallel play.

100. School refusal in midchildhood occurs as an isolated problem often.

Answers

....

94. False: This is acting out.

95. False

96. False: It is a structural error (e.g. adding–ed to say)

97. False: It is the tendency for male and female children to play in same-sex groups.

98. True

99. False

100. False: It occurs with many other social avoidance problems.

101. Twins generally attain puberty later than the non-twins.

102. Adolescent crisis mostly ends with the identification of a dependable figure.

103. Empty nest syndrome is classically due to retirement from job.

104. Anticipatory grief is always cumulative.

105. Freud failed to explain 'punishing' dreams.

106. Secondary autonomous ego functions defend against in-stinctual drives under stress.

107. A transitional object displaces mother as an attachment fig-ure.

Answers

101. True

102. False: The move from dependency to independence is more useful.

103. False: It occurs when the youngest child is about to leave home.

104. False: It can decrease or increase with time.

105. False: He explained it summoning a wish for punishment on the dreamer's part.

106. False: They get autonomous from their initial drive reduction goals.

107. False: It serves to replace her, instead.

108. Overcompensation is a mature defense.

109. Peak experience is the constant, static and final achievement of self-actualizers.

110. Henry Murray proposed personology.

111. Infants serve as a source of security for most mothers.

112. Cognition replaces affect in rationalization.

113. Suppression is just a minor form of repression.

114. Abused children more often use aggression for coping.

115. Abused children have friends who are generally elder than them.

Answers

....

108. True: It is building up of desired traits.

109. False: It is an episodic, brief sense of heightened understanding and euphoria.

110. True

111. False

112. False: This is intellectualization.

113. False: Retrievable forgetting is suppression.

114. True

115. False

116. Spousal abuse dips down during third trimester of pregnancy.

117. In Rorschach one card is colourless.

118. Chaining is linking set of responses to facilitate complex procedures.

119. Child is a responsive-interactive-being from birth itself according to Winnicott.

120. Authority orientation occurs in the phase of conventional morality of Kohlberg.

121. Transsexualism in middle childhood is a normal phenomenon.

122. Most children under five years describe traumatic dreams vividly.

Answers

....

116. False: Very high risk in this period.

117. False: 5–coloured; 5–not coloured.

118. True: A response becomes the stimulus for the second response.

119. True: So it structures the environment actively.

120. True

121. False: It represents an extreme aberration of gender identity.

122. False: Only one fifth can do that.

123. CAMCOG gives score out of 104.

124. The Timberlawn studies initiated research of families as dynamic systems.

125. IQ is directly related to the prevalence of psychiatric disorders.

126. Motor development is cephalocaudal.

127. An older woman is at higher risk of being labeled hysterical than younger woman if both are histrionic.

128. Establishing ego-integrity is the core maturational task of an adolescent.

129. In BASDEC all true answers score one point each.

Answers

....

123. True: It is a comprehensive test for cognition.

124. True

125. False: There is an inverse relationship in fact.

126. True

127. False: It is less likely.

128. False: It is seen in later life.

129. False: Suicidality and hopelessness carry two points each.

130. Older people often fail to handle loss effectively.

131. It is possible to identify temperamental characteristics in first few weeks of life.

132. Blind children are more susceptible to psychiatric disorders than the deaf.

133. Attachment behaviour is characterized by proximity seeking.

134. Massed practice is a procedure to decrease unwanted behaviour.

135. In extinction an initial spurt of behaviour can occur.

136. Token economy is based on response cost method.

Answers

....

130. True: This is against the popular belief that experience in handling losses is protective.

131. True: But stability is variable over time.

132. True

133. True

134. True: It is a form of satiation–employed in tics.

135. True: It is safe to ignore this.

136. True: Tokens for the desired and fines for the unwanted behaviours.

137. Ambiguous cues can disturb repetition of already learnt behaviour.

138. Children from large families demonstrate lower reading achievements.

139. Youngest child in a family suffers a slightly greater risk of school refusal.

140. Infants usually form only one attachment.

141. Boys suffer more than girls due to parental divorce.

142. Guided participation is gradual imitation after careful observation.

143. Time out is easier and equally effective in adolescents than younger children.

Answers

....

137. True

138. True

139. True

140. False: Many may exist, though mother is the primary figure.

141. True

142. True: This is a form of modeling.

143. False: Larger child resists physical removal and adolescents rebel more vigorously.

144. Anhedonia precludes success of CBT in depression.

145. Systemic family therapy employs a circular questioning around an evolving hypothesis.

146. Holding therapy is proposed for Autism.

147. Absence of social achievement in childhood provokes GAD or depression directly.

148. Resilience refers to individual differences in response to social difficulties.

149. Penetrance is an all or none genetic phenomenon.

150. Reinforcement occurs sequentially from last act in backward chaining.

Answers

....

144. True

145. True

146. True: Its efficacy is unproven but.

147. False: Absence of good peer relation is directly provocative but.

148. True

149. False: Incomplete penetrance is possible.

150. True: It can be employed in toilet training.

Psychopathology

1. Freud proposed his theory of paranoid delusion based on 'Memories of My Mental Illness' by Daniel Schreber.

2. Identification is an important mechanism for ego development.

3. Loss of self orientation marks the onset of delirium in hepatic encephalopathy.

4. Organic orderliness is a form of loss of flexibility in delirium.

5. Melting face illusion occurs in panic disorder.

6. Phosphenes are elementary visual hallucinations.

7. Under inclusion is seen in anankastic personalities.

Answers

....

1.   True

2.   False: It is important for superego development.

3.   False: Loss of orientation to time, place, person and self follows in that order in most of the deliria.

4.   True

5.   False: It occurs in hallucinogen abuse.

6.   True: They occur when occipital cortex is stimulated.

7.   True

8. Rumination is the mental state seen at times during a panic attack.

9. Alexithymia is a feature of PTSD.

10. Syllogomania is compulsive filth collecting.

11. Porropsia is a part of macropsia wherein objects gradually enlarge and get nearer.

12. 'Sperrung' is a sudden thought and motor block.

13. Cryptamnesia is seen in late Alzheimer's.

14. Double orientation is seen in chronic schizophrenia.

15. Xenophobia may be seen in atypical depression.

Answers

....

8.   True

9.   True

10. True

11. False: It is a type of micropsia where size of objects is retained but they get retreated!

12. True

13. False: It is seen in early part of the disease. Quotes are employed in speech without remembering their origin from the memory.

14. True: It is the separation of belief from feeling and action.

15. True: Mood reactivity and rejection sensitivity are also seen.

16. Cocooning is strange noise produced during manic episodes.

17. Hallucinations deny a diagnosis of delusional disorder.

18. Amphitryon delusion is a delusional misinterpretation.

19. Magnan's symptom is noted in cocaine intoxication.

20. Most common cause of ageusia is zinc deficiency.

21. In Dorian Gray delusion, an old patient thinks all except him are ageing rapidly.

22. Wednesday evening society was a Christian movement to help parents of psychotic children.

Answers

....

16. False: Severe psychomotor retardation with isolation seen in geriatric depression is called cocooning.

17. False: Tactile or olfactory hallucinations congruent with the delusion may be present.

18. True: It is seen in Capgras's syndrome where spouse is replaced by an identical impostor. In Sosias delusion apart from the spouse other close acquaintances are also replaced.

19. True: It is also called formication.

20. False: It is depression.

21. True: Dorian Gray is Oscar Wilde's creation.

22. False: It was the Vienna psychoanalytic society started by Freud's students.

23. Strephosymbolia is also called delusional perception.

24. Flagellation is masochistic or sadist pleasure of whipping.

25. Ataraxia is lack of any disturbance in thought.

26. Obsessive ruminations are often philosophical questions achieving bizarre conclusions.

27. Obsessions secondary to dementia are strongly resisted.

28. Monolithic systems are characteristic of anankastic thinking.

29. The disaster image affects compulsive cleaners.

30. Procaine infusion causes visual hallucinations.

Answers

23. False: It is the revere reading seen in dyslexia.

24. True

25. True: It is an ancient Roman psychotherapy. Tranquilizers were called ataractics for some time.

26. False: They are pseudophilosophical and they achieve no conclusions at all.

27. False: The element of resistance is usually absent in dementia.

28. True: This is a tendency to make judgments which mean the same thing inspite of diverse presenting problems.

29. False: It affects compulsive checkers.

30. True

31. Ribot introduced the term alexithymia.

32. In poverty of speech patient may speak much.

33. Motor neglect is tested by clock drawing test.

34. Most common delusions in dementia are grandiose delusions.

35. Kraus coined the term hypernomia.

36. Meticulously imitated voices are found difficult to be discriminated from hallucinations by psychotic patients.

37. Picture sign in dementia is a hallucination of talking portraits.

Answers

....

31. False: He introduced anhedonia. Alexithymia was introduced by Sifneos.

32. True: In poverty of thought speech is always less. But here there may be much speaking but full of stock phrases and repetitions so actually very little is 'said'.

33. False: Visual neglect can be made out. Buttoning a shirt makes motor neglect obvious.

34. False: Persecutory delusions are the commonest.

35. True: It is the exaggerated adaptation to social norms seen in premorbid personality of some depressed patients.

36. False: They do this easily.

37. False: It is a delusional belief that individuals on television are present in the house.

38. Malignant narcissism is the infiltration of aggression into the pathological self.

39. It is impossible to overcome pseudohallucinations voluntarily.

40. *Gedankanlautwerden* is a transition between vivid imagination and auditory hallucination, according to Schneider.

41. Devaluation is a defense mechanism used by borderline personalities.

42. Anomie results in weakened community relations.

43. Transition from elementary to complex hallucinations may be due to increased affective involvement.

Answers

....

38. True: The pathological self is usually grandiose here, leading to antisocial behaviour at times.

39. False: According to Jaspers, it can be overcome with difficulty.

40. True

41.   False: It is seen in narcissistic personalities. Splitting is the core coping strategy in narcissism but.

42. True

43. True: This is Klosterkotter's view.

44. Staring at a whitewall increases likelihood of visual hallucinations during alcoholic delirium.

45. 'Depressio sine depressione' stands for depression with prominent somatic symptoms of anxiety.

46. Pathological lying is a feature of narcissism.

47. Obsessive patients show distorted adaptation to social norms.

48. Siege experience is a derealization phenomenon.

49. Coenaesthetic sensations are seldom reported spontaneously by patients.

50. Drug induced and innate hallucinations cannot be distinguished by schizophrenic patients usually.

Answers

44. True: Optical hallucinations of fine structures (hairs, webs, threads) are common.

45. True: Simply- somatoform depression.

46. True

47. True: This is called dysnomie sometimes.

48. False: It is a combination of multiple delusions and hallucinations seen in organic psychoses usually.

49. True: These misperceptions usually fluctuate with stress.

50. False: They often successfully discriminate them.

51. Psychomotor retardation is accompanied by a change in perception of time.

52. Inability to distinguish wishes from reality is a feature of mania not depression.

53. Sense of confusion can occur in mania.

54. In fantasy thinking the subject is completely unaware of the mood, affect or drive which motivates it.

55. For delusions the most important criterion is impossibility of their contents.

56. Delusions are communicated as explanations usually.

57. Psychological irreducibility is a feature of primary delusions.

Answers

....

51.   True: Depressed patients thus overemphasize on their past.

52.   False: This is common for both. It results in poor decision making.

53.   True: This is the boiling over of mania.

54.   False: Though the process is non-goal directed, the subject may be aware of the force behind.

55.   False: This is not the case always. E.g. Out of sociocultural context and in delusions of jealousy.

56.   False: They are expressed as judgments usually.

57.   True: They are often the first events in psychopathological processing.

58. Loosening of associations enhances concrete thinking.

59. Mythomania occurs in histrionic personality disorder.

60. Autoscopy is a somatic perceptual experience.

61. Attributing coenaesthetic hallucinations to external agents may herald the onset of schizophrenia.

62. In depression there is difficulty in thought termination.

63. Excessive abstract thinking cannot occur in schizophrenia.

64. Dysarthria occurs in schizophrenia.

65. Delusional memories are false memories with no correlating past events.

Answers

58. True: This may be due to DLPFC lesions leading to dysfunctional working memory.

59. True: Also called pseudologia fantastica.

60. False: It is a visual perceptual experience.

61. True: Klosterkotter stressed this point.

62. True: So ruminations with negative themes may occur.

63. False: It can occur, again due to working memory defects.

64. True

65. False: They may be either false memories without past events or distorted memories interpreted with delusional meaning.

66. Crowding of thoughts is also known as thought acceleration.

67. Verbigeration is seen in agitated depression.

68. *Vorbeireden* is seen in schizophrenia.

69. Cryptographia is a feature of private thought symbolism.

70. In double phenomenon two conflicting parts are experienced at the same time.

71. Delusional atmosphere usually gives rise to certainity of self reference.

72. Cognitive schema disappears totally after recovery from acute depressive episode.

Answers

66. False: Crowding is a disturbance in control of thought–a variant of thought insertion.

67. True: Also in organic disorders and schizophrenia.

68. True: Also in Ganser's syndrome, organic disorders and hysteria.

69. True: Neologisms and cryptolalia are other features.

70. True: This differentiates it from the multiple personality disorder.

71. True: This later becomes fully evolved with specific delusional meanings.

72. False: It becomes latent–to be reactivated by later stressful events.

Questions

73. Pseudologia fantastica is fantasy thinking with complete exclusion of reality.

74. Disordered awareness of boundaries of self is always psychotic.

75. The content of dysmorphophobia is a delusion usually.

76. Disturbance of body image usually extends to inanimate objects too.

77. Temper tantrums are minor signs of affect dysregulation.

78. Striving for autonomy is a frequent feature in personality of bipolar patients.

79. Depersonalization in mood disorders is usually of delusional intensity.

Answers

73. False: Complete exclusion leads to autistic withdrawal. Limited exclusion is seen in hysteria and some delusions too.

74. False: It can occur in ecstatic states too.

75. False: It is an overvalued idea usually.

76. False: And surprisingly height is often perceived normally.

77. True: Akiskal has been emphasizing this.

78. True: Unconventional and norm-giving behaviours are also described.

79. False: This may be true in schizophrenia.

Questions

80. Hyperschemazia is obsessive concern over arrangement of objects.

81. Agreeing for treatment implies complete insight.

82. Confabulation can occur without primary memory disturbances.

83. Overinclusion is a disorder of flow of thought.

84. Mannerisms can be conspicuous expressions involving objects.

85. Imaginative thinking is always goal-oriented and non-pathological.

86. Alcoholic palimpsests produce subjective uneasiness.

Answers

80. False: It is a pathological accentuation of body image due to organic lesions.

81. False: Not necessarily true always.

82. False: It is always secondary to memory deficits.

83. False: It is due to failure to preserve conceptual boundaries e.g. schizophrenia.

84. True: e.g. Peculiar dressing pattern with a particular delusional meaning is also a mannerism.

85. False: It becomes pathological if the subject attaches more weight to his representation of events than other possible interpretations.

86. False: Here the faded memory is patched up by layers of other events usually.

87. Déjà vu is a paramnesia.

88. Muddling is extreme tangentiality with superadded pressure of speech.

89. Memory disturbances are common in mood disorders.

90. Mania a potu is a twilight stage.

91. Incoherent thinking in delirium is clinically similar to derailment.

92. Imageries are the most common perceptual disturbances in oneiroid states.

93. 'The Interpretation of Dreams' is the first book authored by Freud.

Answers

87. True

88. False: Extreme fusion with derailment constitutes muddling.

89. False: Though there are often complaints about impaired memory, no deficit is found in objective tests.

90. True

91. True

92. False: Multiple scenic hallucinations are the most prominent features.

93. False: He coauthored 'Studies on Hysteria' with Breuer, four years before this book.

94. Freud observed that hypnosis was much more successful with the lower classes.

95. Loosening of association is a positive formal thought disorder.

96. Contents of oneiroid state are often remembered.

97. 'The psychology of dementia praecox' is written by Emil Kraeplin.

98. Technical neutrality is essential for applying psychoanalysis in therapy.

99. Projection is more mature than projective identification.

100. In exhibitionism, compulsive nature of behaviour is strong.

Answers

....

94. True

95. True: It leads to abnormal concepts.

96. True: This differentiates it from twilight state.

97. False: It was first published by Jung. This made Freud to invite Jung to Vienna.

98. True: Merton Gill proposed this.

99. True: In projection there is no longer any emotional contact with what is projected.

100. True

101. Delusional mood accompanies delusional atmosphere.

102. Preexisting organic pathology is often found in pathological intoxication.

103. Working through is the repeated elaboration of an unconscious conflict during psychoanalysis.

104. 'Containing' was described by Winnicott.

105. Pseudocyesis is a disorder of woman.

106. In schizophrenia there is loosening of link among elements in experience of time.

107. Schizophrenic hallucination is passive and defenseless.

Answers

....

101. True: It is an 'internal set' correlating with 'external atmosphere'.

102. True

103. True: It is a major task for the analyst.

104. False: 'Holding'—The capacity of analyst to withstand emotionally any primitive transference, was his concept. Bion described containing.

105. False: It can occur in men too, especially in schizophrenia or cerebral syphilis.

106. False: This occurs in mania (Binswanger).

107. True: In alcoholic hallucination, active perception with localization, identification and action occurs (Zutt).

108. Endokinesis is the process of changing from normality to depression following stress.

109. Disintegration anxiety is the most primitive form of anxiety.

110. Diaschisis is a sudden reversible clinical phenomenon that cannot be explained anatomically.

111. Chronogenetic localization stands for unfolding of neuropsychiatric functions over time.

112. Morel proposed the degeneration theory of psychiatric etiology.

113. Neuropsychological approach to psychopathology was introduced by Greisinger.

114. Delusional atmosphere is part of the process that underlies all primary delusional phenomena.

Answers

....

108. True: This occurs in typus melancholicus (Tellenbach).

109. True: Kohut proposed this. It is a fear of falling apart.

110. True: Von Monakow's concept.

111. True: This is a part of dynamomorphological concept in neuropsychiatry. So processes are better localized using time (kinetic melody) than the anatomical address.

112. True

113. False: Wernicke made this important contribution.

114. True

115. Ephebolia is a perverse sexual interest on adolescents.

116. Exhibitionism without masturbation is accompanied by aggressive feelings towards others.

117. Power struggle between parent and child becomes evident first in feeding behaviour.

118. Stereotypes are always abnormal.

119. Delusional misidentification is based on delusional percept.

120. Most pedophiles do not have interest in adult sex.

121. *Doppelganger* is phenomenologically related to Capgras's syndrome.

Answers

115. True: It is similar to pedophilia.

116. True

117. True: This leads to feeding disorder if severe.

118. False: Some occur in normal development as motor exercises.

119. True

120. False: Generally there is a mixed interest.

121. False

....

122. Possession states occurring in schizophrenia have clear consciousness.

123. Apocalyptic experiences of visions are usually eidetic imageries.

124. Opposition in motor act is equivalent to thought block in speech.

125. In paraphilias, individual deviance has the lowest risk of psychiatric symptoms.

126. Couvade syndrome occurs only in husbands of pregnant women.

127. A pseudohallucination has a quality of ideas rather than perceptions.

128. Aggression reduces pain perception.

Answers

122. True: In contrast dissociative possessional states demonstrate disturbed consciousness.

123. False: They are most likely to be pseudohallucinations.

124. False: Obstruction is the correct equivalent.

125. False: It carries high risk of ostracism, alienation and psychiatric morbidity.

126. False: It is less frequently described in other family members also.

127. True: This holds for imagery too.

128. True: So in war fields, wounds are less painful.

129. Perplexity is a feature of early stages of delusion formation.

130. Thought blocking occurs in depression.

131. Obsessive avoidance is more due to fear of consequences than the actual confrontation.

132. Negativism is a passive process of poor cooperation in catatonia.

133. Delusional atmosphere may not be specific for schizophrenia.

134. Either mutism or akinesis is seen in stupor.

135. Epileptic automatism is common in initial episodes of seizures and later it extinguishes

Answers

129. True: This gets relieved when a particular delusion is fully formed from preceding delusional atmosphere.

130. True

131. True: The opposite is true in phobic avoidance.

132. False: It is an active process of resisting all attempts to make contact.

133. True: Janzarik's structural — dynamic coherence concept allows this possibility. (Ref: Oxford textbook)

134. False: Both should be seen together to qualify as stupor.

135. False: It is more common in chronic epileptics.

136. Information is processed largely in semantic form.

137. Change in affect influences speed of thought.

138. Circumstantiality occurs in mental retardation.

139. Memories cannot occur as obsessions because of lack of senselessness.

140. Phobic and anankastic states often occur together.

141. In polarized delusions the delusional reality is intermingled with actual facts.

142. Stock phrases have idiosyncratic meaning and are rarely repeated by the patient.

Answers

136. False: It is either iconic or echoic; semantic form is synthe-sized later.

137. True

138. True: Also in organic disorders and schizophrenia.

139. False: The memory may be sensible in its content, but not the context. At times this may be unpleasant and terrifying too.

140. True

141. True

142. False: By definition, stock phrases are repeated throughout conversation.

143. Locating depression as a bodily sensation is a first rank equivalent.

144. Ekbom's syndrome most commonly occurs as a part of affective psychosis.

145. Depersonalization is a rare symptom.

146. Heymans coined the term derealization.

147. In dissociation there is loss of consciousness.

148. Unlike other forms of hysteria, mass hysteria occurs commonly in young boys.

149. Frigophobia is a phobic disorder with morbid fear of cold.

150. Affect is preserved in depersonalization experiences.

Answers

....

143. True

144. True: It can also occur as a separate delusional disorder and in organic states.

145. False: After depression and anxiety, depersonalization is the most frequent psychiatric symptom (Stewart, 1964).

146. False: Mapother used it first in 1935.

147. False: To be exact, there is narrowing of consciousness with amnesia.

148. False: Young girls are the most vulnerable.

149. False: It is an obsessive-compulsive state with fear of cold—seen in East Asia.

150. False: Any mental function may or may not be the subject of this change, but affect is invariably involved (Ackner, 1954).

Psychopharmacology

Questions

1. Tyramine reaction can be treated with β blockers only.

2. Thyroxine acts on cholinergic receptors to convert antidepressant nonresponders to responders.

3. Haloperidol has a narrow therapeutic index.

4. Fluoxetine causes discontinuation reaction.

5. Fluoxetine is sometimes useful to treat akathisia.

6. Abrupt withdrawal of levodopa can cause NMS.

7. Bon bon sign is seen in tardive dyskinesia.

8. Tremors are the most common neurological adverse effects of TCAs.

Answers

1.   False: Sometimes calcium channel blockers can be useful.

2.   False: It acts on ß receptors to bring this effect.

3.   False

4.   False: Imipramine and SSRIs with brief $t_{1/2}$, given for long course in high doses cause discontinuation reaction frequently.

5.   False: Fluoxetine itself can cause akathisia.

6.   True

7.   True: It is a type of lingual movement similar to sucking a candy.

8.   True

9. Velnacrine is a prodrug of tacrine.

10. Salbutamol ameliorates lithium induced tremors.

11. Promethazine can cause false positive pregnancy test.

12. Diazepam is a metabolite of chlordiazepoxide.

13. IM lorazepam is the drug of choice for amphetamine induced agitation.

14. Benzodiazepine withdrawal can mimic multiple sclerosis.

15. Carbamazepine can replace benzodiazepine during withdrawal of the latter.

16. Carbamazepine can cause hyponatremia.

Answers

....

9.   False: Velnacrine is the leucopenia inducing metabolite of tacrine.

10. False: ß blockers are useful but.

11. True

12. True

13. False: Lorazepam is used in all substances induced agitation except amphetamine.

14. True: With ataxia, paresthesia and fasciculations, it mimics multiple sclerosis often.

15. True: Carbamazepine acts on peripheral benzodiazepine receptors.

16. True: It acts on vasopressin 2 receptors.

17. Antidepressant drugs are not effective in chronic fatigue syndrome.

18. Sertindole is limbic selective dopamine antagonist.

19. TCA withdrawal can cause extrapyramidal symptoms.

20. Topiramate potentiates $GABA_B$ receptor.

21. Lithium can produce transient stuttering.

22. Antipsychotics are the first line drugs in Lewy body dementia.

23. Phenothiazines are the sedatives of choice in acute intermittent porphyria.

Answers

17. False: Mirtazapine is particularly effective.

18. True

19. True

20. False: $GABA_A$ potentiation.

21. True: Lithium induces delirium, occurring with level more than 1.5 mEq/L, is heralded by stuttering, lethargy and fasciculations.

22. False: They worsen functional capacity further.

23. False: Chloral hydrate should be used. Also avoid barbiturates and benzodiazepines.

24. Amphetamine induced psychosis has prominent thought disorder.

25. Depressed schizophrenia patients are more sensitive to extrapyramidal side effects of antipsychotics.

26. Increasing concentration of alcohol intoxicates more than decreasing concentrations in blood, given the same blood levels.

27. Bruxism is an adverse effect of amphetamine.

28. Cannabinoids can be used to treat muscular spasms.

29. Cannabis intoxication leads to tachypnea and respiratory failure.

30. LAAM is a widely abused opioid substance.

Answers

....

24. False: It has predominant visual hallucinations and few or no thought disturbances.

25. True

26. True: This is called the Mellanby effect.

27. True

28. True: They can be utilized in muscle spasm related to multiple sclerosis.

29. False: Cannabis intoxication has no effect on respiratory rate and it never causes death by itself.

30. False: LAAM (l-α-acetyl methadol) is an opioid substitute given once in 2 days, unlike once daily methadone.

31. Nomifensine is a norepinephrine–dopamine reuptake inhibitor.

32. GABA$_B$ agonist baclofen can induce depression.

33. Naltrexone can treat self injury in the mentally retarded.

34. Modafinil is a α_1 antagonist used in narcolepsy.

35. Acamprosate acts by facilitating GABA and inhibiting glutamate.

36. Chlorpromazine has a single metabolite molecule.

37. Sertindole is promoted for acute negative symptoms.

38. Meprobamate is a nonbenzodiazepine anxiolytic.

Answers

31. True: It can be used for depression in Parkinsonism or epilepsy.

32. False: It can cause mania.

33. True

34. False: It is a α_1 agonist.

35. True

36. False: More than 100 are demonstrated.

37. True

38. True: It is a muscle relaxant too. It interacts with GABA-BDZ complex without binding to GABA receptor.

39. ECT can be used to treat NMS.

40. Preferred preanesthetic medication for ECT is glycopyrrolate.

41. Postictal arrhythmias are more common after methohexital anesthesia in ECT.

42. Haloperidol accelerates learning in autistic children.

43. Lithium is contraindicated in ADHD.

44. School phobia is an adverse effect of haloperidol.

45. Pimozide aggravates somatic delusions.

46. Amoxapine is the least sedating conventional antidepressant.

Answers

....

39.   True

40.   True: But avoid if heart rate is more than 90.

41.   False: Thiopentone predisposes to this adverse effect.

42.   True

43.   False: Lithium is sometimes useful in treating ADHD.

44.   True: Especially when used for childhood tics.

45.   False: It is the drug of choice in somatic delusions. E.g. dysmorphophobia.

46.   False: Desipramine is the least sedating.

47. Thioridazine causes hyperkalemia.

48. ECT has no danger of manic switching.

49. All antidepressants have the same response rate when given singly.

50. Theophylline increases fluvoxamine levels in blood.

51. Meperidine causes hyperkalemic crisis in patients taking MAO_A inhibitors.

52. Befloxatone is a potential MAO_B blocking antidepressant.

53. Antibulimic effects of SSRIs occur earlier than antidepressant effect.

Answers

....

47. False: It causes hypokalemia.

48. False

49. True: The line can be drawn at 67% responders in 8 weeks and 33% nonresponders throughout.

50. False: The opposite via CYP 1_{A2} inhibition is true.

51. True

52. False: It is a RIMA like moclobemide, in its early developmental phase.

53. True: It needs higher than usual antidepressant dose.

54. SSRIs target the terminal axonal reuptake system directly.

55. Fluoxetine inhibits NO synthase.

56. Reboxetine produces dry mouth by anticholinergic actions.

57. Sustained release preparations provoke seizure less frequently than immediate release bupropion.

58. Dopamine reuptake inhibitors are potentially addictive.

59. Tramadol inhibits serotonin and norepinephrine reuptake.

60. Venlafaxine produces dose dependent increase in antidepressant efficacy.

Answers

....

54. False: Now it has been recognized that somatodendritic $5HT_{1A}$ receptors are the earliest targets in whose locality reuptake is first inhibited, leading to synaptic increase in 5HT levels after desensitization.

55. False: Paroxetine inhibits NO synthase.

56. False: It causes pseudoanticholinergic syndrome by augmenting noradrenaline transmission.

57. True

58. True: They can act on reward pathway to cause addiction.

59. True: It is a kappa agonist used for pain relief.

60. True: This is absent in other antidepressant drugs.

61. Lithium is effective in 65% of bipolar patients.

62. Lamotrigine inhibits carbonic anhydrase.

63. Topiramate can cause weight gain.

64. Pindolol is a 5HT 1A partial agonist.

65. TCAs act faster and better than benzodiazepines in GAD.

66. Tryptophan depletion worsens response to SSRIs in OCD.

67. Fluoxetine produces weight gain through 5HT2C antagonism.

68. Trazadone is extremely sedating.

Answers

61. False: Lithium is effective in only 40–50%.

62. False: Topiramate is the correct choice.

63. False: It is unique among proposed mood stabilizers, causing weight loss, not gain.

64. True: It is a ß blocker that can augment SSRIs similar to buspirone by $5HT_{1A}$ partial agonism.

65. False: They act slower but better than benzodiazepines.

66. False: This may apply to depression not OCD.

67. False: It produces weight loss by $5HT_{2C}$ agonism.

68. True: via H_1 block.

69. St John's wort may be teratogenic.

70. Gabapentin inhibits GABA reuptake.

71. Tianeptine acts on peptide neurotransmission to produce antidepressant effect.

72. Clonazepam has a lesser abuse potential.

73. OCD needs higher dose of antidepressants to start with.

74. Flumazenil is an inverse agonist in panic disorder patients.

75. Benzodiazepines are widely used in PTSD.

76. All serotonin dopamine antagonists reduce prolactin levels.

Answers

....

69. True: It can cause spermic mutation.

70. True

71. False: It enhances 5HT reuptake.

72. True: Due to longer $t_{1/2}$.

73. False: Same starting but higher maintenance dose and longer interval for onset.

74. True: Benzodiazepine receptor set point shifts in panic disorder.

75. False: They carry a high abuse potential and find limited use hence.

76. False:

77. Loxapine has conventional antipsychotic properties.

78. Quetiapine inhibits cholesterol synthesis in lens.

79. Ziprasidone inhibits serotonin and norepinephrine reuptake.

80. Fluvoxamine increases risk of seizures with clozapine.

81. Risperidone has no active metabolites.

82. Sertindole resembles serotonin structurally.

83. Sertindole was temporarily withdrawn due to reported hepatotoxicity.

84. Methylphenidate reverses the direction of dopamine transporter.

Answers

....

77. True: But it is a SDA

78. True: But demonstrated in lower animals — not sure in humans.

79. True: It may act as potential anxiolytic. It has $5HT_{1A}$ agonist property too.

80. True: Via $CYP1_{A2}$ inhibition.

81. False: Risperidone has an active atypical antipsychotic metabolite.

82. True

83. False: It was due to QTc prolongation.

84. True: Thus it facilitates dopaminergic transmission.

85. L-amphetamine is highly selective for dopamine transporter.

86. Stimulants act preferentially at mesocortical pathway.

87. ADHD patients exhibit higher abusive potential for stimulants.

88. Rivastigmine is highly selective for butylcholinesterase.

89. Metrifonate inhibits RBC acetylcholinesterase.

90. Galantamine directly activates nicotinic receptors.

91. Acetyl-l-carnitine is an acetylcholine analogue.

92. Piracetam is a glutamate derivative.

Answers

85. False: It inhibits both norepinephrine and dopamine transporter.

86. True: In low doses this selectivity is exhibited.

87. False: Peculiarly they show no tolerance or reverse tolerance and so, lower abuse potential on chronic usage.

88. False: It acts more on acetyl cholinesterase.

89. True: RBC monitoring can predict brain enzyme activity.

90. True: This is apart from its acetyl cholinesterase inhibition.

91. True: It resembles acetylcholine structurally.

92. False: It is a GABA derived nootropic.

Questions

93. Low initial response predicts high risk for alcohol / stimulant abuse.

94. Cocaine produces respiratory stimulation.

95. Reverse tolerance can develop after single high dose cocaine use.

96. Hyperphagia can occur in cocaine withdrawal.

97. Amphetamines produce more intense euphoria than cocaine.

98. MDMA acts by mimicking serotonin.

99. MDMA produces a total lack of empathizing ability.

100. All hallucinogens are $5HT_{2A}$ agonists.

Answers

93. True: May be due to poverty of receptors leading to defective internal reward system.

94. False: High dose depresses respiratory centre.

95. False: It develops after chronic use only.

96. True

97. False: The euphoria is less intense but longer lasting.

98. False: It releases serotonin.

99. False: MDMA intake increases sense of empathy.

100. True

Questions

101. Phencyclidine is both a stimulant and depressant.

102. PCP produces rotational nystagmus.

103. Marijuana increases accuracy of time perception.

104. Depersonalization can occur in cannabis abusers.

105. Cannabis does not produce tolerance or dependence.

106. Nicotine temporarily inactivates the nicotinic receptors.

107. Naltrexone is prescribed for first 180 days of alcohol abstinence.

108. H1 antagonism is the best correlate for weight gain due to antipsychotic drugs.

Answers

....

101. True

102. False: It produces vertical nystagmus usually.

103. False: It produces loss of temporal awareness.

104. True: It is a part of amotivational syndrome.

105. False: It produces tolerance. Dependence is well demonstrated in animal studies.

106. True: This causes 'minirush'.

107. False: First 90 days — highest relapse rate.

108. True: False: Loxapine has no effect on weight.

109. Loxapine produces weight loss.

110. ß agonists reduce leptin secretion.

111. Dopaminergic agents boost NO synthetase.

112. Tamoxifen induced depression responds well to SSRIs.

113. Progesterone causes excitotoxic destruction of dendritic spines in late luteal phase.

114. Cyclical progesterone administration is less depressing than regular use.

115. Anticholinergics carry abuse potential.

116. High blood glucose postpones onset of tardive dyskinesia.

Answers

109. **True**

110. True

111. True: Apomorphine is a candidate to increase arousal response.

112. False: It is usually difficult to treat.

113. True: It destroys all those spines that sprouted during early phase under estrogenic influence.

114. False: Vice versa is true.

115. True: They can be misused for their euphoric effect.

116. False: Diabetes, affective disorder and female sex are risk factors.

117. NMS is usually accompanied by severe / moderate hyperthermia.

118. Ziprasidone is a weight neutral antipsychotic.

119. Antipsychotic usage is a risk factor for DVT.

120. Same dose of Aripiprazole is to be used in each psychotic episode.

121. Trifluoperazine is the most sedative of phenothiazines.

122. Risk of agranulocytosis increases with duration of clozapine use.

123. Sulpiride is D2 selective in low doses.

124. Risperidone produces first dose effect.

Answers

....

117. **False:** Mild fever is common.

118. True

119. True

120. True: 15 mg every time. But data is limited.

121. False: It is the least sedative phenothiazine.

122. False: Highest risk in first 18 weeks. After a year risk is same as any neuroleptic.

123. False: D_4 selective at low doses and D_2 selective in higher doses.

124. True: BP monitoring and titrated dosage is necessary.

125. Amisulpiride is useful to substitute diabetogenic antipsychotics.

126. Fluphenazine depot preparation should be avoided if depressive features are florid.

127. Sulpiride can augment clozapine.

128. Risperidone decreases plasma clozapine levels significantly.

129. Clozapine induced nocturnal enuresis warrants discontinuation of the drug.

130. Dose reduction can ameliorate clozapine induced myocarditis.

131. Mianserin may be effective in akathisia.

Answers

125. True: It has no effect on GTT.

126. True

127. True

128. False: It augments clozapine by increasing its level.

129. False: Manipulation of dose schedule is all that is needed.

130. False: This warrants stopping clozapine once for all.

131. True: Cyproheptadine and mianserin are serotonin antagonists and are useful in akathisia.

132. Osteoporosis is linked to antipsychotic usage.

133. Antipsychotics sensitize leptin receptors.

134. Topiramate produces weight gain.

135. Intermittent usage of lithium worsens bipolar disorder.

136. Lithium is effective in steroid induced psychosis.

137. Topiramate can produce cognitive decline.

138. Carbamazepine should not be used within 14 days of MAO inhibitor usage.

139. Abnormal LFT is acceptable when using carbamazepine.

Answers

132. True: Due to hyperprolactinemia.

133. False: They increase leptin levels by desensitizing receptors, leading to obesity.

134. False: It is a potential weapon against drug induced weight gain.

135. True: But this is untrue in unipolar depression.

136. True

137. True

138. True: It resembles TCAs structurally.

139. False: This may indicate an ongoing hypersensitivity warranting drug withdrawal.

140. Lithium induced nephrogenic diabetes insipidus is irreversible.

141. Stimulants are useful in OCD.

142. Valproate produces pancreatitis.

143. Citalopram is the safest SSRI in QT_c prolongation.

144. Low dose anticonvulsants are useful in alcohol withdrawal.

145. Desipramine is the most rapid anxiolytic among antidepressants.

146. Toxic dose of lithium produces fine tremors.

147. Carbamazepine may produce toxicity with flu vaccine.

Answers

140. False: Usually it is reversible. In long term users(>15 years) it is irreversible.

141. True: They are effective in predominant obsessive impulses.

142. True

143. False: All SSRIs except citalopram are safe in QTc prolongation.

144. False: Usually high dose carbamazepine is needed. But this is intolerable for most patients.

145. False: It has no effect over anxiety symptoms.

146. False: In therapeutic range fine tremors occur; in toxic dose coarse tremor is seen.

147. True: But this is not proven.

148. Aripiprazole has site-selective action according to dopamine availability.

149. Omega 3 fatty acids are useful to augment clozapine in mania.

150. In children lithium is effective in lower range of therapeutic limit.

Answers

148. True

149. False: They may benefit neurodegeneration in schizophrenia.

150. False: Adolescents and children need higher serum levels.

Section 5

Psychiatric Disorders

1. Postcardiotomy patients form the single largest group of hospitalized patients with delirium.

2. Knife blade gyri are seen in Pick's disease.

3. Language and memory are often preserved in Huntington's dementia.

4. Negative correlation exists between schizophrenia and rheumatoid arthritis.

5. ICD10 can label a patient to have schizophrenia earlier than DSM IV

6. Pain threshold is raised in autistic children.

7. Suicide is the commonest cause of death in PTSD[1].

1 PTSD – Post Traumatic Stress Disorder.

Answers

....

1. False: Patients with alcohol withdrawal form the single larg-
    est inpatient group with delirium.

2. True

3. True

4. True

5. True: ICD 10 requires one month of symptoms only. DSM
    requires 6 months with atleast one month active symptoms.

6. True: Both pain and fever threshold are elevated.

7. False: Suicide rates are no more than normal population in
    PTSD.

8. Hereditary basal ganglia calcification mimics positive symptoms.

9. According to DSM IV a manic episode should last at least 1 week necessarily.

10. Acceleration of thought is not subjectively experienced by the patient.

11. Marriage protects males but not females against major depression.

12. Vigilant task execution is affected in schizophrenia.

13. Tardive dyskinesia worsens under stress.

14. Bipolar disorder has lower suicide rate than schizophrenia.

Answers

8. **False:** Fahr's disease mimics negative symptoms.

9. **False:** Duration does not matter if symptoms warrant hospitalization.

10. False: Subjective racing of thoughts can occur.

11. True

12. True

13. True

14. False: 15% in bipolar against 10% in schizophrenia.

15. Hypersexuality is the characteristic feature of Kluver Bucy syndrome.

16. 20% of Wilson's disease presents with psychiatric symptoms.

17. Gaze aversion is a feature of fragile X syndrome.

18. Mesial sclerosis is the commonest cause of complex partial seizures.

19. Demyelination at centrum semiovale is noted in Binswanger's disease.

20. Anomic aphasia can occur as a side effect of TCAs.

21. ALS[2] can present with dementia alone.

2 ALS – Amyotrophic Lateral Sclerosis

Answers

....

15. **False:** It may be true in animals. In man inappropriate sexual comments are noted (Trimble et al); Frank hypersexuality is rare.

16. True

17. True

18. True

19. True

20. True

21. True

22. Alzheimer's dementia is associated with migrainous head-ache.

23. Self injurious behaviour is seen in neuroacanthocytosis.

24. Myoclonus is seen in dialysis dementia.

25. Mania occurs in Huntington's disease.

26. Cataplectic attack is usually precipitated by fatigue.

27. Automatic behaviour is often seen in narcolepsy.

28. Narcoleptic attacks are most frequent in mornings.

29. Bedwetting is more common in NREM stage.

30. Head banging may be normal in infants.

Answers

....

22. False: CADASIL – Cerebral Autosomal Dominant Arteriopathy with Subcortical Infarcts and Leukoencephalopathy is migraine associated but.

23. True

24. True

25. True

26. False: Strong emotions are the common triggering factors.

27. False: Seen in one third only.

28. False: Afternoon is the worst period for them.

29. True: But it can occur in any stage.

30. True: Occasional head banging is common.

31. Sense of terror is often recalled in *pavor nocturnus*.

32. In nocturnal panic attack, patients fall back to sleep almost immediately.

33. Febrile illness increases the frequency and intensity of nightmares.

34. Insomnia may occur in narcolepsy.

35. Bland euphoria occurs without hyperactivity in SLE[3].

36. Hyperthyroidism causes psychomotor retardation in elderly.

37. Mania is common in endogenous Cushing's syndrome.

3 SLE – Systemic Lupus Erythematosus.

Answers

....

31. True: But no dreams or imageries are clearly recalled.

32. False: Trouble sleeping again is a useful diagnostic feature here.

33. True

34. True

35. False: It is seen in multiple sclerosis.

36. True: This is apathetic hyperthyroidism.

37. False: It is common in exogenous origin of disease.

38. Sensory tics do not occur in Tourette's syndrome.

39. Abulia can be differentiated from akinesia using close supervision.

40. Akathisic impulses increase on standing up.

41. Patients may become mute in akathisia.

42. Restless legs syndrome induce marching in place.

43. Acquired stutterers suffer equal block with first or subsequent syllables.

44. Anorexia nervosa is associated with family history of OCD.

45. Conduct disorder is the most common comorbid diagnosis in ADHD.

Answers

38. False: An itch or premonitory urge is frequent.

39. True: Abulic patient responds to supervision with relative alacrity.

40. False: They come down by standing.

41. True: It is due to buzzing thoughts defying expression.

42. False: This is a feature often seen in akathisia.

43. True: Developmental stutterers frequently have an easy second syllable.

44. True: Also to GAD, depression, obsessive compulsive personality disorder and eating disorders in the family.

45. False: 35% ADHD patients have oppositional deviance and 26% conduct disorder.

46. Diltiazem can cause akathisia.

47. Extreme compliance as a childhood temperament is related to anorexia nervosa.

48. ADHD vanishes in majority by adolescence.

49. Mental fatigue is essential to diagnose chronic fatigue syndrome.

50. Lower premorbid intellect is a risk factor for Alzheimer's disease.

51. Patients with Lewy body dementia have better life expectancy than Alzheimer's.

52. The Hamilton Depression Rating Scale is not ideal to measure outcome in older patients.

Answers

46. True: But this is very rare.

47. True: Also perfectionism and negative self evaluation.

48. False: 70% ADHD children continue to have it by adolescence and 65% adolescents with ADHD are troubled in adulthood too.

49. False: CDC criteria do not insist on this symptom. Oxford criteria insist but.

50. True: Head injury and Down's are other risk factors.

51. False: 6 years average against 7–10 years.

52. True: It includes several somatic items that may turn false positive in this group.

53. Family history of alcohol abuse worsens the prognosis of bulimia.

54. Better therapeutic response is noted in ADHD with comorbid problems than pure ADHD patients.

55. Earlier the onset, better the prognosis in anorexia nervosa.

56. Women are more prone than men for CFS[4].

57. Manganese deficiency is demonstrated in CFS.

58. BMI[5] matched to population weight is the most used outcome measure in anorexia nervosa.

59. Many behavioural problems in dementia resolve spontaneously in short term.

4 CFS – Chronic Fatigue Syndrome
5 BMI – Body Mass Index

Answers

53. False: Surprisingly this is linked to good prognosis. Higher social class and younger age are other favourable factors.

54. True: Ref: Swanson GM et al. *J Am Acad Child Adol Psychiatry* 2001; 40; 168–79.

55. True

56. True: Relative risk is 1.3 to 1.7

57. False: Magnesium is the culprit. IM magnesium may be better than placebo in CFS.

58. False: Morgan Russell scale is the most used outcome measure.

59. True: But using antipsychotics increased the percentage of responders.

60. Reminiscence therapy relies on recent memory.

61. Bibliotherapy is advising people to read case histories of recovered patients.

62. Improving bone mineral density reduces fracture in anorexia nervosa.

63. CFS may be associated with hormone mediated hypotension.

64. Childhood depression is typically acute or subacute.

65. 10–15% older people meet DSM IV criteria for depressive disorder.

66. Prevalence of learning disabilities diagnosed using IQ scores is 1%.

Answers

60. False: It relies on remote memory; relatively preserved in mild to moderate dementia.

61. False: Usually 'feel good' written materials (like motivating books) are prescribed.

62. False: No correlation to this effect by HRT is demonstrated.

63. False: Neurally mediated hypotension is a proposed mechanism.

64. False: It is often insidious.

65. False: 10–15% old people have depressive symptoms not disorder.

66. False: Prevalence is around 3% if only IQ is a criterion. By stricter definition there is only 1% prevalence.

67. GAD[6] remits spontaneously in a significant number of patients.

68. Deliberate self harm is noted in congenital pain insensitivity.

69. The recurrence rate of depression is similar in adults and children.

70. People with eating disorders can alternate between the diagnosis of bulimia and anorexia nervosa.

71. In autism sleep latency is short.

72. Infrequent vocalization is the earliest symptom but goes unnoticed in Tourette's syndrome.

73. Episodic course is common in initial years of OCD.

Answers

67. **False:** Spontaneous remission is very rare.

68. **False:** Accidental self injury, not DSH is seen.

69. **True:** 70% in 5 years.

70. **True**

71. **False:** Many autistic children show problems in sleep initiation.

72. **False:** Vocalization starts years after motor tics.

73. **True:** Later it becomes chronic.

74. Panic disorder is associated with increased suicides.

75. There is a higher occurrence of early menarche in patients with eating disorders.

76. Fear of contamination responds well to CBT[7].

77. Negative interpretation of stressful life events is a causal factor for GAD.

78. Copropraxia is a feature of Tourette's disorder.

79. 25% reduction in YBOCS[8] score indicates clinical improvement in most of the trials.

80. Insidious onset schizophrenia responds better to treatment than acute onset.

7 CBT – Cognitive Behavioural Therapy
8 YBOCS – Yale Brown Obsessive Compulsive Scale.

Answers

74. False: Attempted suicides may be more but.

75. True: Physical or sexual abuse, low self esteem, mood disorder and perfectionism are also highly prevalent.

76. True: Also overt ritualistic behaviour.

77. False: This is implicated in panic disorder but.

78. True: It is involuntary obscene gesturing.

79. True: Some use 35% mark.

80. False

81. Prodromal periods of cognitive impairment precede the onset of vascular dementia.

82. Braak and Braak staging is used in neuritic plaque identification.

83. Frontal white matter abnormalities correlate strongly with depression in dementia.

84. Diffuse Lewy body dementia is more common in women.

85. Severe OCD responds better to SSRIs than mild/moderate OCD.

86. In very advanced dementia, several neuropsychiatric symptoms occur.

87. REM sleep behaviour disorder is common in diffuse Lewy body dementia.

Answers

81. True: These transient vascular cognitive impairment periods are similar to TIAs.

82. False: A CERAD (Consortium to Establish Registry for AD) criterion is for neuritic plaques; Braak and Braak's criterion is for neurofibrillary tangles.

83. True

84. False: Men have higher risk.

85. True: Also later onset with no previous drug treatment predicts good response.

86. False: In advanced cases the severe disability masks behavioural changes or neuropsychiatric symptoms.

87. True

88. Narcissistic individuals are often the first child in their families.

89. Lack of empathy is a feature of histrionic personality.

90. Subjective distress is a prerequisite to diagnose personality disorders.

91. CSF ß amyloid protein is elevated in Alzheimer's.

92. Lewy bodies in vagal nucleus can produce isolated dysphagia.

93. Chronic pain can be accompanied by a profound personality change.

94. Brief psychotic episodes occur in paranoid personality disorder.

Answers

....

88.   True

89.   False: Empathizing ability is present in histrionics.

90.   False: Either subjective distress or social/occupational mal-
      functioning is sufficient.

91.   False: ß amyloid is decreased while tau protein is increased.

92.   True

93.   True: The algogenic psychosyndrome.

94.   True: This occurs during stress.

Questions

95. There is a higher prevalence of chronic tics and Tourette's disorder in relatives of girls than boys with Tourette's.

96. Childhood pica is increased in houses with pets.

97. In dementia, executive dysfunction has the highest correlation with neuropsychiatric symptoms.

98. Rumination disorder is often linked to major developmental delays.

99. In DSM IV feeding disorder is diagnosed with height as a criterion.

100. Primary enuresis is strongly associated with conduct disorder.

101. Korsakoff patients cannot learn new things.

....

95. True: This gender threshold effect is also seen in ADHD.

96. True: Imitation may play a role.

97. True: This marks DLPFC involvement.

98. False: This is true only in 25%

99. False: Weight is the criterion.

100. False: Secondary enuresis demonstrates such association.

101. False: They learn but they are unable to remember the process of learning.

102. In cortical dementia abnormal movements may occur.

103. Circuit related syndromes affect instrumental functions in dementia.

104. Errorless procedures facilitate learning in amnesia.

105. Obsessional content is not related to the prognosis of OCD.

106. Penetration is necessary to induce pain in dyspareunia.

107. Antisocial behaviour gradually increases with age.

108. Borderline personality disorder does not have an operational criterion in ICD-10.

Answers

....

102. True: But this is rare; usually myoclonus.

103. False: They affect fundamental functions like emotion, motivation, execution etc. Instrumental functions are affected in signature syndromes like aphasia, apraxia etc.

104. True: Also in dementia this helps.

105. True

106. False

107. False: It decreases gradually.

108. True: It is the only disorder of its kind to be so.

109. Dysprosody is the commonest language disorder in Alzheimer's.

110. During rumination (merycism) the infant is often restless and perplexed.

111. Cannabis psychosis remits on complete abstinence.

112. There is always some frontal involvement in Korsakoff's syndrome.

113. Behavioural inhibition occurs during late worsening stage of social phobia.

114. 'Quiet vagina' is an extended start-stop technique.

115. Incidence of frontotemporal dementia increases with advancing age.

Answers

....

109. False: Anomia progressing to transcortical sensory aphasia is the characteristic defect. FTD[9] has dysprosody usually.

110. False: The infant looks quiet without any discomfort.

111. True: But cannabis induced schizophrenia has its own course.

112. True: This is a prerequisite for confabulation.

113. False: This may be an early expression of social phobia.

114. True: Here, with female astride, male partner gets desensitized to the warm sensation of vagina.

115. False: Peak incidence occurring in sixth decade, no further increase with age is seen.

....

9 FTD – Fronto Temporal Dementia

Questions

116. Hypercholesterolemia is a risk factor for Alzheimer's.

117. Psychomotor activity is lethargic in schizoid personality disorder.

118. A strong genetic factor is demonstrated in functional enuresis.

119. Throughout the life span a female predominance in OCD is demonstrated.

120. Premature ejaculation occurs within 15 seconds from the beginning of intercourse.

121. Transcortical motor aphasia is the most common language disturbance in Crutzfeld-Jacob disease

122. Palipsychism is preservation and superimposition of mental activities normally processed sequentially.

Answers

116. True: Cholesterol increases amyloid protein production or aggregation.

117. True: It lacks gesture and rhythmic movement.

118. True

119. False: Boys are more affected in adolescence.

120. True: This is an ICD 10 statement.

121. True

122. True: It occurs in anterior thalamic infarction as a part of vascular dementia.

123. Froment's sign is noted in Parkinsonism.

124. Prebedtime agitation is a feature of conduct disorder.

125. Applied tension is employed in treating blood-injury-injection phobia.

126. Hysteria is common in families with antisocial personality disorder.

127. Antisaccade test is a measure of orbital frontal function.

128. Trans-entorhinal cortex is the initial site of neurofibrillary tangles formation.

129. Quinacrine is effective against prion proteins in vitro.

130. Rumination can be an infantile form of self stimulation.

Answers

123. True: Marked loss of limb tone when contralateral limb is actively moved — in cases with minimal rigidity especially.

124. False: It may be a presentation of separation anxiety disorder.

125. True: Paradoxical parasympathetic arousal is seen in this specific phobia.

126. True: Genetic linkage is proposed.

127. False: It measures executive function.

128. True: Neocortex is involved only in advanced phases. But frontal and limbic cortex are least affected by neuritic plaques.

129. True: Thorazine also has this property.

130. True: Other self stimulatory behaviours are also commonly associated.

131. Yielding to compulsions quickens recovery in OCD.

132. Selective mutism is not associated to social phobia.

133. In reactive attachment disorder unusual emotional involvement towards a stranger may be present.

134. In Heidenhain variant of CJD frank psychosis is common.

135. Aggression is frequent feature of schizoid personalities.

136. Separation anxiety disorder cannot be diagnosed after 7 years of age.

137. Children with selective mutism are often perfectly normal in biological development.

138. Panic disorder has a shorter course in males.

Answers

131. False: It is a poor prognostic factor.

132. False: 97% of selectively mute patients show social phobia.

133. True: This is seen in disinhibited type only. In inhibited type, lethargy, depression and disinterest are common.

134. False: Visual disturbances presenting as perceptual disorder progressing to cortical blindness is common.

135. False: They are infrequent.

136. False: Up to 18 years we can diagnose this (DSM IV).

137. False: Around one third have a language disorder and one half show speech development problems.

138. False: Though uncommon in males, they suffer longer but with lesser risk of agoraphobia / depression

139. Psychosis is more common in frontotemporal dementia than Alzheimer's.

140. Children with encoperesis have a longer colonic transit.

141. Overcorrection is the most effective technique in treating stereotypic movement disorder.

142. Man made disasters produce higher rates of PTSD than natural ones.

143. Obsessional slowness and concern with symmetry are predominant in males.

144. 'La belle indifference' is seen only in hysteria.

145. Artistic talent may emerge after developing dementia.

Answers

139. False: Depression is also less in FTD.

140. True: Especially if constipation is associated.

141. True: Psychostimulants may aggravate the stereotypies.

142. True

143. True

144. False: It is a nonspecific sign.

145. True: Especially in FTLD–semantic dementia and primary progressive aphasia, this is noted.

146. In speech phobic type of selective mutism, there is no motivation to overcome the problem.

147. In obsessional fear, patients actively seek fear provoking stimuli to avoid them.

148. Identity diffusion is a central problem in borderline personality disorder.

149. Histrionic personalities have difficulty making friends.

150. Symptomatic gambling occurs secondary in to depression.

151. Long delays are common in diagnosing narcolepsy.

152. Jetlag syndrome does not produce chronic sleep disturbances.

Answers

146. False: Often they show strong motivation.

147. True: But this is absent in phobia.

148. True

149. False: They make easy friends; but fail to sustain the relationship often.

150. True: This is one of the five varieties of pathological gambling.

151. True

152. False: It may become chronic in frequent travelers.

153. Insomnia is more prevalent in men.

154. Tics in Tourette's syndrome disappear in sleep.

155. Suicide is usually preceded by years of suicidal behaviour.

156. Compulsive buying is the most common impulse control problem in psychiatry OPD.

157. Majority of suicides in schizophrenia occur immediately after recovering from an acute exacerbation.

158. Insufficient sleep syndrome has a strong biological basis.

159. Pathological gamblers have higher than normal risk of attempting suicide.

Answers

153. False: It is more common in women.

154. False: Frequently they do persist in NREM 1 & 2 stages.

155. True

156. True: Intermittent explosive disorder comes next.

157. False: They occur during an active phase usually.

158. False: It is purely occupational and personality based.

159. True: Eight times more.

160. Idiopathic insomnia is a disease of geriatric patients usually.

161. Lethality of first suicidal attempt is higher in males.

162. Affective symptoms most commonly accompanied impulsive acts in episodic dyscontrol.

163. Lifetime prevalence of OCD increases with age.

164. When hypochondriasis has unilateral symptoms it is predominantly left sided.

165. In compensation neurosis remarkable improvement after financial settlement is the rule.

166. Daytime sleep episodes are refreshing in narcolepsy.

Answers

....

160. False: It begins typically in childhood.

161. True

162. True: The most common symptoms are manic-like irritabil-ity, racing thoughts and increased energy.

163. False: This may be due to increased incidence recently or recall bias.

164. True

165. False: Family support is more influential in recovery than financial gain.

166. True

167. Need for symmetry predicts poor prognosis in OCD.

168. Vague wandering with loss of identity is seen in fugue.

169. In hypochondriasis the main concern is symptom relief.

170. In Ondine's curse breathing control is normal in wakefulness.

171. Childhood stealing is more common in OCD patients than the normal population.

172. Manic stupor develops slowly compared to the sudden onset in psychogenic stupor.

173. In adjustment disorder, presence of anhedonia is determined by the severity of perceived stress.

Answers

167. True: So does male sex and early onset.

168. False: Purposeful behaviour under new identity character-izes fugue. Vague wandering is seen in psychogenic amne-sia.

169. False: The concern is the reassurance that he does not have any particular major disease. Somatizing patients are sat-isfied with symptom relief but.

170. True: During sleep, apnoeic episodes occur.

171. False

172. True

173. False: Anhedonia is conspicuous by its absence in adjust-ment disorder.

174. Acute gastric dilatation occurs in anorexia nervosa.

175. Nocturnal seizure is the commonest cause of sleep related injury.

176. Insight oriented therapy is very useful in intermittent explosive disorder.

177. Cataplexy is often partial not total loss of muscle tone.

178. Drugs reducing periodic limb movements improve associated daytime sleepiness.

179. OCD is the most common comorbidity with kleptomania.

180. Hanging is the commonest mode of suicide globally.

181. Axis II disorders are often seen in Klein-Levine syndrome.

Answers

174. True

175. False: Sleep terrors / somnambulism top the list.

176. False: CBT with anger management strategies are the most useful.

177. True: It presents as sudden inability to articulate or strange feeling in the face, unlocking of the knees etc.

178. False: There is no evidence to this effect.

179. False: Mood disorders esp. bipolar are the commonest.

180. True

181. False

182. Chasing of losses indicate loss of control over gambling.

183. Hypnagogic hallucinations characteristically evoke no response from the subject.

184. Among the depressed, hopelessness is the best predictor of suicide.

185. Immigrants entering western culture have a higher rate of suicide than the host culture.

186. Compulsive buying is classified in DSM IV not ICD10.

187. Sleep terrors are more common than sleep walking.

188. In trichotillomania hair pulling from other persons can occur.

Answers

....

182. **True**

183. **False:** They may frighten so much that the subject guards with weapons or pets in the room.

184. True

185. False: Though higher than original culture, it is lesser than the hosts.

186. False: Both systems do not entertain this as a separate diagnosis.

187. False

188. True: E.g. from spouse, doll, children etc.

189. Hypercarotenemia is seen in anorexia nervosa.

190. Poor sleep in narcoleptics usually improves with age.

191. Anorexia nervosa evolves into depressive disorder in significant number of patients.

192. A bulimic binge diet is usually low in protein.

193. Sleep walking adults often show complete amnesia for the episode.

194. Obsessional behaviour may be normal in childhood only.

195. Trichotillomania is egosyntonic.

196. Sleep drunkenness is a hallmark of idiopathic hypersomnia.

Answers

189. **True**

190. False: There is no tendency to improve usually.

191. False: No such trend is reported.

192. True: 'Carbohydrate craving' is not consistently proved but.

193. False: Children are totally amnesic; adults recall dream like mentation often.

194. False: It may be normal in all ages.

195. True

196. False: It is seen only in poly-symptomatic but not mono-symptomatic variant.

....

197. Bulimic patients seek voluntary treatment more often than anorexia nervosa patients.

198. Emotional instability in the first week of puerperium may be a risk factor for subsequent depression.

199. Irritability is the most frequent mental symptom in Klein-vine syndrome.

200. Idiopathic hypersomnia is more common than narcolepsy.

201. In trichotillomania, hair pulling is pursued inspite of pain.

202. 10–15% of parasuicide patients go on to commit suicide.

203. ECT has moderate antiobsessional effect.

Answers

....

197. True: The distress associated with bulimic episodes is a possible cause.

198. True

199. True: A feeling of unreality comes next.

200. False: Only one for every ten patients with narcolepsy.

201. False: Typically it is painless.

202. True

203. False: It has no specific effect evident against obsessions.

204. Mood instability is maximum on the fifth postpartum day in postpartum blues.

205. Mild learning disability is clustered in lower socioeconomic classes and severe cases in upper classes.

206. Automatic hair pulling is compulsive in nature.

207. Nocturnal eating behaviour is associated with excessive thirst.

208. Serotonin partial agonist (mCPP) challenge produces mild euphoria in patients with impulse control disorder.

209. Postsynaptic $5HT_{2A}$ receptor density is increased in suicide victims.

210. Elevated urinary cAMP is noted in postpartum blues.

Answers

....

204. True

205. True: Blackie et al in 1975 demonstrated this in a Scottish study.

206. False: Focused hair pulling is more compulsive. 75% of trichotillomaniacs are primarily automatic.

207. False: No hunger, thirst or purging behaviour is seen.

208. True

209. True: This may be a compensatory response to decreased presynaptic binding.

210. True: Significance is not known.

211. The tremor of GAD worsens with intention.

212. REM sleep behaviour disorder is closely associated with Parkinsonism.

213. Avoidant behaviour is noted in trichotillomania.

214. Low blood cholesterol is associated with increased suicidality.

215. Depressive mood precedes the syndrome of brain fag.

216. Deep diaphragmatic breathing is common in hyperventilation syndrome.

217. Sleep efficiency gets reduced with normal ageing.

218. Restless legs occur exclusively during sleep.

Answers

211. True: It is present at rest too.

212. True

213. True: Situations revealing hair loss are avoided.

214. True: This may be mediated by decreasing serotonin function.

215. False: Depression is usually reactive to academic failures here.

216. False: High thoracic breathing is common rather.

217. True

218. False: It can occur in any period of inactivity, e.g. watching TV.

Questions

219. Scalp biopsy has no role in trichotillomania.

220. In Down's, the extent of mosaicism parallels the extent of abnormal dermatoglyphics.

221. P[300] latency increases with age in both Down's and normal people.

222. A peculiar tip toe gait is seen in autism.

223. Sleep disturbance is present in most cases of PSP[10]

224. Mental retardation if associated with Neurofibromatosis is profound.

225. Patau's syndrome is associated with increased maternal age.

10 PSP – Progressive Supranuclear Palsy.

Answers

....

219. False: Biopsy can pick the difference between compulsive hair pulling and other skin conditions.

220. True

221. True: But marked increase in this latency occurs prematurely in Down's patients.

222. True: This mimics the gait seen in equinovarus deformity.

223. True

224. False

225. True: Also true for Edward's syndrome.

226. Cognitive speed in mental retardation increase with each episode of mania.

227. Autistic behaviour improves substantially in children with psychosis.

228. A child often gets injured during temper tantrums.

229. Short lasting nocturnal dystonia is a form of epilepsy.

230. Nonaccidental injury is higher in smaller families.

231. In autism an advanced phase of language development may be revealed when speech is begun.

232. Most school refusers have good academic attainments.

Answers

....

226. False

227. True: Other symptoms of childhood psychosis may remain unchanged but.

228. False: Others may be injured–but self injury is rare.

229. True: This is increasingly being appreciated of late.

230. False

231. True: This never occurs in other developmental disorders.

232. True

233. Charles Bonnet syndrome is visual hallucination linked to poor vision in the elderly.

234. Eccentricity of personality is a marked feature of Diogenes syndrome.

235. Anorexia nervosa occurs more commonly in diabetes.

236. Self injurious behaviours are more likely to be serious in blind children.

237. Specific reading disorder is the most common learning disability among conduct disorder patients.

238. Autistic children use peripheral vision more than central vision.

239. School refusal in adolescence is relatively benign.

Answers

233. True: Insight is more or less preserved here.

234. False: Even physical illness, dementia or other psychiatric illnesses can cause senile squalor syndrome.

235. True: So does bulimia nervosa.

236. True

237. True

238. True: So they perceive moving objects better.

239. False: It is more pathological than childhood school refusal.

240. Repetitive absconding in conduct disorder may be a suicidal equivalent.

241. Plagium is child stealing.

242. Child stealing is commonly committed by women.

243. Father daughter incest is the most common incest.

244. Indecent exposure is the commonest sexual offence.

245. Catatonic symptoms are more common in interictal psychosis.

246. Agitation is a prominent symptom in hypopituitarism.

247. Temporal lobe dysfunction is common among sexual deviants.

Answers

240. True

241. True

242. False: Men are common offenders.

243. True

244. True: It is the one with the best prognosis too.

245. False

246. False: Apathy is quite common but.

247. False: It is low.

248. In ecmnesic hallucinations, memories are vividly recalled and relived with greater intensity.

249. Complex partial status is commoner than absence status.

250. Children with temporal lobe EEG spikes have low neuroticism than those with generalized spikes.

251. Childhood schizophrenia is more common in boys than in girls.

252. Amphetamine-induced psychosis is usually clinically distinguishable from schizophrenia.

253. Formication is a recognised feature of cocaine abuse.

254. Cocaine-induced psychosis is typically short-lived.

Answers

248. True

249. False

250. True: But aggression is more.

251. True

252. False: Usually indistinguishable.

253. True: Formication ('cocaine bugs') refers to the sensation of insects crawling under the skin.

254. True

255. Amphetamine is a psychedelic drug.

256. The acute ingredient in 'magic' mushrooms is LSD.

257. Personality disintegration is seldom seen in monosymptomatic delusional disorders.

258. Duration of at least 1 month is required for an ICD-10 diagnosis of 'persistent delusional disorder'.

259. HIV infection is a recognised cause of persistent delusional disorder.

260. The litigious subtype of paranoid personality disorder is also known as querulous paranoia.

261. When a psychotic patient commits homicide, the victim is usually a stranger.

Answers

255. False

256. False: Psilocybin.

257. True

258. False: At least 3 months.

259. True

260. True

261. False: Usually a family member.

262. Schizophrenia is more common in the learning disabled population.

263. Schizophrenia is associated with an increased density of cortical $5HT_{2A}$ receptors.

264. Neuropathological changes are seldom seen in schizophrenic patients presenting with their first psychotic episode.

265. Patients with schizophrenia are more likely to develop Alzheimer's disease than non-schizophrenics.

266. In schizophrenia, acute onset of symptoms has a significantly better prognosis than an insidious onset.

267. Placebo response in schizophrenia is negligible.

Answers

....

262. True

263. False: Decreased density of $5HT_{2A}$ and increased density of $5HT_{1A}$ receptors in the cortex.

264. False: Reduced brain volume and dilated ventricles are commonly seen in first-episode patients.

265. False: No such link.

266. True

267. False: At least a third show some improvement.

268. Micrographia is a typical feature of antipsychotic-induced Parkinsonism.

269. Clozapine reduces the risk of suicide in schizophrenia.

270. Acute myocarditis due to clozapine is associated with eosinophilia.

271. Leonard introduced the concept of 'cycloid psychoses'.

272. Pathological jealousy typically has a chronic course.

273. Intermetamorphosis is a delusional misidentification syndrome.

274. In shared delusional disorders, *folie simultanee* is more common than *folie imposee*.

Answers

....

268. False: Micrographia is much less common in drug-induced Parkinsonism than in idiopathic Parkinsonism.

269. True

270. True

271. True

272. True

273. True: Other delusional misidentification syndromes include Capgras, Fregoli and the syndrome of subjective doubles.

274. False: It is other way round.

275. In erotomanic delusional disorder, both the patient and the patient's object of affection typically come from the same socio-economic group.

276. Executive functioning is likely to be affected in chronic schizophrenia.

277. DSM-IV criteria for schizophrenia are broadly based on Schneiderian first-rank symptoms.

278. Phencyclidine (PCP) causes an acute psychosis.

279. In alcoholic hallucinosis, the voices are usually in the third person.

280. Alcoholic hallucinosis responds poorly to neuroleptics.

281. Alcoholic hallucinosis occurs in clear consciousness.

Answers

....

275. False: The object of affection is usually of higher socio-economic status.

276. True

277. False: ICD-10 criteria are broadly based on first-rank symptoms.

278. False: PCP is also called 'angel dust'.

279. False: Usually in the second person.

280. False: In most cases, the response is rapid and complete.

281. True

282. Temporal lobe epilepsy is a recognised cause of acute psychotic symptoms.

283. Fregoli syndrome is also known as 'illusion of doubles'.

284. Hypochondriacal delusions are characteristic of depressive psychoses.

285. Insight is poor in patients with body dysmorphic disorder.

286. 'Camouflaging' is a feature of body dysmorphic disorder.

287. The effect of life events is greater in precipitating depressive episodes than in precipitating schizophrenic episodes.

288. Agenesis of the corpus callosum is more common in schizophrenics than in controls.

Answers

....

282. True

283. False: Capgras syndrome is known by this name.

284. True: Also nihilistic delusions.

285. True

286. True: Refers to the patient attempting to hide their 'defect' by excessive make-up, wearing hats, etc.

287. True: Although life events play a role even in schizophrenia.

288. True: Cavum septum pellucidum, aqueduct stenosis and A-V malformations are also more common in schizophrenics.

Questions

289. In patients with schizophrenia, there is a decreased P300 latency.

290. Akathisia induced by antipsychotics is a significant risk factor for suicide.

291. Schizophrenia has an earlier age of onset in females than in males.

292. Schizophrenia is significantly more common in females than in males.

293. Insidious onset of symptoms is a poor prognostic factor in schizophrenia.

294. Suicide in schizophrenics typically occurs several years after the onset of the illness.

Answers

....

289. False: Increased latency.

290. True

291. False: The other way around.

292. False: It is equally common in males and females.

293. True: Other poor prognostic factors include male sex, presence of negative symptoms, co-morbid personality disorder / substance abuse, earlier age of onset and long duration of untreated illness.

294. False: Typically occurs in the first few years of the illness.

295. Schizophrenia is more common in those born in winter.

296. High expressed emotion (EE) significantly increases the risk of relapse in schizophrenia.

297. Schizophrenia has an incidence of 1% per year.

298. Overinclusive thinking is a feature of schizophrenia.

299. Schizophrenia is more common in the unmarried.

300. 'Residual schizophrenia' is a subtype included in both ICD-10 and DSM IV.

301. First-rank symptoms are pathognomonic of schizophrenia.

Answers

....

295. True

296. True: High EE includes hostility, critical comments and over-involvement.

297. False: The incidence is about 20 per 100,000 per year. The lifetime risk is about 1%.

298. True: First described by Cameron. It refers to the inability to maintain conceptual boundaries.

299. True

300. True

301. False: They also occur in affective and organic psychoses.

302. Catatonic schizophrenia is equally common in different parts of the world.

303. The concept of hebephrenia was first introduced by Hecker.

304. Dilated lateral ventricles on neuroimaging are a feature of chronic schizophrenia.

305. The prognosis of schizophrenia is the same across the world.

306. Perplexity is a characteristic feature of acute schizophrenia

307. The commonest subtype of schizophrenia is paranoid schizophrenia.

308. Kasanin introduced the concept of catatonia.

Answers

302. False: More common in developing countries.

303. True

304. True

305. False: The prognosis is better in developing countries.

306. True

307. True

308. False: Kasanin described 'schizoaffective psychosis' while Kahlbaum first described catatonia.

309. Presence of grandiose delusions excludes a diagnosis of schizophrenia.

310. ICD-10 requires duration of 6 months or more for a diagnosis of schizophrenia.

311. Schizophrenia is more common in the lower socio-economic classes.

312. Co-morbid substance abuse significantly increases the risk of suicide in schizophrenia.

313. In simple schizophrenia there are no positive symptoms.

314. Brown and Harris conducted the pioneering study looking at the role of EE in schizophrenia.

315. An increase in parahippocampal volume is a neuropathological finding in schizophrenia

Answers

309. False: Grandiose delusions typically occur in mania, but can also occur in schizophrenia and organic psychoses.

310. False: ICD-10 requires 1 month and DSM IV requires 6 months.

311. True: Not clear whether poverty is a cause or effect.

312. True

313. True

314. False: They conducted the pioneering study on the role of social factors in depression.

315. False: A decrease is seen.

316. Monosymptomatic delusional disorder has a significantly better prognosis than schizophrenia.

317. An ICD-10 diagnosis of simple schizophrenia requires duration of at least 2 years.

318. An ICD-10 diagnosis of schizotypal disorder requires duration of at least 2 years.

319. Hebephrenia is a schizophrenic subtype in both ICD-10 and DSM IV.

320. In schizophrenia, first-rank symptoms do not have prognostic significance.

321. Crow proposed the distinction of schizophrenia into reality distortion, psychomotor poverty and disorganization subtypes.

322. In schizophrenia, the suicide risk is about 1%.

Answers

316. True

317. False: 1 year.

318. True

319. False: Only in ICD-10.

320. True

321. False: Liddle proposed this.

322. False: About 10%.

323. Dementia is more common in paraphrenia patients.

324. Simple schizophrenia was first described by Kraepelin.

325. Hebephrenic schizophrenia is characterised by an excellent prognosis.

326. Hebephrenic schizophrenia is characterised by a fatuous affect.

327. Neuropathologically, schizophrenic brains are smaller and lighter than the brains of normal controls.

328. The prevalence of schizophrenia in urban areas is greater than in rural areas.

329. Schizotypal disorder was first described by Kendler.

330. In schizophrenic patients, the production of interleukin-2 is increased.

Answers

....

323. False: The incidence is not much different.

324. False: By Bleuler.

325. False: Poor prognosis.

326. True

327. True

328. True

329. True

330. False: Decreased.

Questions

331. The risk of schizophrenia in the offspring of 2 schizophrenic parents is about 25%.

332. Maternal infection with influenza during pregnancy is associated with schizophrenia in the offspring.

333. The monozygotic concordance in schizophrenia is 5%.

334. The concept of 'double bind' communication is associated with Bateson.

335. According to Bleuler, apraxia was a fundamental feature of schizophrenia.

336. Presence of hallucinations and delusions excludes a diagnosis of hebephrenic schizophrenia.

337. In ICD-10, schizotypal disorder is included under 'Disorders of adult personality and behaviour'.

Answers

331. False: About 50%.

332. True: Particularly 2nd trimester infection.

333. False: About 50%.

334. True: Refers to the child being given contradictory, mutually exclusive messages. Was postulated in the 1950s as an aetiological factor for schizophrenia.

335. False: Bleuler's fundamental symptoms of schizophrenia were autism, affective incongruity, ambivalence and loosening of association.

336. False: ICD-10 (category F 20.1) states that 'hallucinations or delusions must not dominate the clinical picture, although they may be present to a mild degree'.

337. False: It is included under 'Schizophrenia, schizotypal and delusional disorders'.

338. For an ICD-10 diagnosis of postschizophrenic depression, the patient must have met the diagnostic criteria for schizophrenia within the past 12 months but should not meet them at the present time.

339. Late-onset schizophrenia like psychosis is more common in females.

340. Bleuler coined the term 'dementia praecox'.

341. Decreased need for sleep is a characteristic feature of mania.

342. Presence of psychotic symptoms is incompatible with an ICD-10 diagnosis of hypomania.

343. ICD-10 requires duration of at least 1 week for a diagnosis of hypomania.

Answers

338. True

339. True

340. False: Kraepelin coined this term. Bleuler coined the term 'schizophrenia'.

341. True

342. True: The diagnosis becomes mania.

343. False: At least 4 days.

Questions

344. Psychotic symptoms in mania are typically mood-incongruent.

345. Bipolar type II disorder is a diagnosis in ICD-10 but not DSM-IV.

346. A diagnosis of rapid cycling bipolar disorder is made when there are at least 6 discrete episodes in a year.

347. One-third of the patients with cyclothymia subsequently develop bipolar affective disorder.

348. Bipolar disorder has a lifetime prevalence of about 0.5%.

349. Bipolar disorder is more common in females.

350. Panic disorder is more common in bipolar patients than in controls.

Answers

344. False: Mood-congruent.

345. False: It is the other way around.

346. False: At least 4 episodes.

347. True

348. True

349. False: Equally common in males and females.

350. True

351. HIV infection is a recognised cause of mania.

352. Alcohol abuse is more common in bipolar patients than in controls.

353. Mania is more common in autumn and winter.

354. The risk of postpartum psychosis is significantly increased if the mother has a history of bipolar disorder.

355. Jet lag is a recognised precipitant of mania.

356. Concordance for bipolar disorder is greater in monozygotic twins than in dizygotic twins.

357. Bipolar disorder has an earlier age of onset than unipolar depression.

Answers

....

351. True

352. True

353. False: More common in spring and summer.

354. True

355. True

356. True

357. True

358. Bipolar I disorder has an earlier age of onset than Bipolar II disorder.

359. The average duration of a manic episode is 4 weeks.

360. In the course of bipolar disorder in one's lifetime, the duration between successive episodes gradually lengthens.

361. In patients with bipolar disorder, the same type of life event can precipitate either mania or depression.

362. Patients with bipolar disorder experience about 10 affective episodes in their lifetime.

363. The overall prognosis of bipolar disorder is poorer than unipolar depression.

364. Bipolar I has a better prognosis than Bipolar II disorder.

Answers

....

358. True

359. False: 4 months.

360. False: Gradually decreases.

361. True

362. True

363. True

364. False: It is the other way around.

365. Acute onset of symptoms is a good prognostic factor in bipolar disorder.

366. Rapid cycling bipolar disorder is more common in males.

367. Rapid cycling bipolar disorder responds better to treatment than the nonrapid cycling variety.

368. In rapid cycling bipolar disorder, bipolar type II is more common than type I.

369. Lithium has been shown to reduce the risk of suicide in bipolar disorder.

370. ECT is contraindicated in acute mania.

371. In the treatment of bipolar disorder, applying cognitive therapy techniques increases compliance with medication.

Answers

365. True

366. False: More common in females.

367. False: It is the other way around.

368. True

369. True

370. False: ECT is a recognised treatment for acute mania.

371. True

372. In general, patients with bipolar disorder experience more depressive episodes than manic episodes in the course of their lifetime.

373. Lithium is particularly effective in rapid cycling bipolar disorder.

374. About 30% of the patients with acute mania respond to lithium within 7 days.

375. Rebound mania is a consequence of abrupt discontinuation of lithium.

376. Hypersomnia is more common in bipolar depression than in unipolar depression.

377. Sodium valproate is superior to lithium in bipolar patients with mixed affective states.

Answers

....

372. True

373. False

374. False: The response rate is about 60% in 7 days, according
      to most studies.

375. True

376. True

377. True

378. In treating bipolar disorder, combining two mood stabilisers provides no additional benefit.

379. Kraepelin first described 'manic depressive insanity'.

380. In ICD-10, cyclothymia is included under 'Disorders of adult personality and behaviour'.

381. For an ICD-10 diagnosis of cyclothymia, the mood instability should have been present for at least 6 months.

382. Mania is a recognised feature of ICD-10 cyclothymia.

383. Dysthymia is more common in females.

384. Alcohol abuse is more common in patients with cyclothymia than in controls.

Answers

....

378. False: This is a treatment strategy that may be useful in resistant patients.

379. True

380. False: It is included under 'Persistent mood (affective) disorders – category F 34.0.

381. False: At least 2 years.

382. False: Then the diagnosis becomes either manic episode or bipolar affective disorder.

383. True

384. True

385. Cyclothymia is more common in the relatives of bipolar patients.

386. Hyperthymia is a diagnosis in ICD-10.

387. REM latency is increased in patients with dysthymia.

388. Bipolar disorder is more common in the upper social classes.

389. Mania is a dose-related side effect of corticosteroids.

390. The risk of suicide in the manic phase of bipolar disorder is negligible.

391. Leonhard pioneered the distinction of affective disorders into unipolar and bipolar categories.

Answers

....

385. True

386. False

387. False: Decreased.

388. False: This had been suggested by earlier studies, but not by later studies.

389. True

390. False

391. True

392. Cyclothymia is more common in males.

393. Hypersomnia is a classical feature of seasonal affective disorder (SAD).

394. Benefit from phototherapy in SAD usually takes 3 to 4 weeks to manifest.

395. SAD is significantly more common in females.

396. Patients with bipolar disorder show deficits in attention even when they are euthymic.

397. In bipolar disorder, there is usually a 2 to 4 day interval between emergence of prodromal symptoms and evidence of full-blown mania.

398. Smoking in bipolar disorder is directly proportional to the severity of the illness.

Answers

....

392. False: Studies have suggested that it is either equally common, or slightly more common in females.

393. True

394. False: Benefit is usually apparent in 3 to 4 days.

395. True: It is about 4 times more common in females.

396. True

397. False: Usually there is a 2 to 4 week interval during which the symptoms get gradually worse, if untreated.

398. True

399. Bipolar disorder is more common in patients with velo-cardio-facial syndrome (VCFS).

400. Obstetric complications are a recognised risk factor for future mania in the offspring.

Answers

....

399. True: Schizophrenia, schizoaffective disorder and ADHD are also more common in VCFS.

400. False:
   1) Post traumatic stress disorder.
   2) Amyotrophic lateral sclerosis.
   3) Systemic upus erythematosus.
   4) Chronic fatigue syndrome.
   5) Body mass index
   6) Generalized anxiety disorder.
   7) Cognitive behavioural therapy.
   8) Yale Brown obsessive compulsive Scale.
   9) Frontotemporal dementia.
   10) Progressive supranuclear Palsy.